PREGNANCY

COOKBOOK

By Trimester

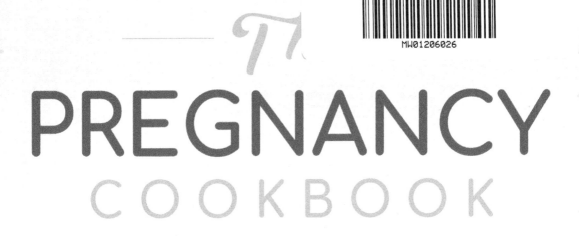

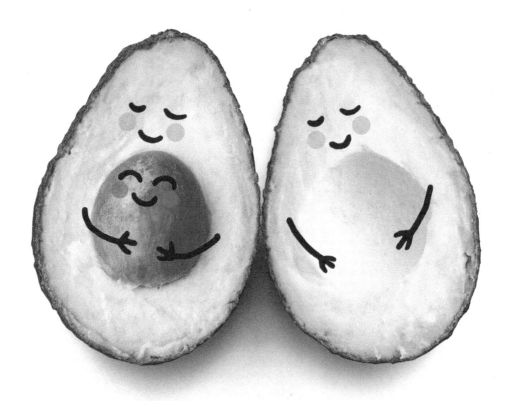

Delicious Recipes, Meal Plans, and Prenatal
Nutritional Guides for You and Your Baby

OLIVIA PHILLIPS

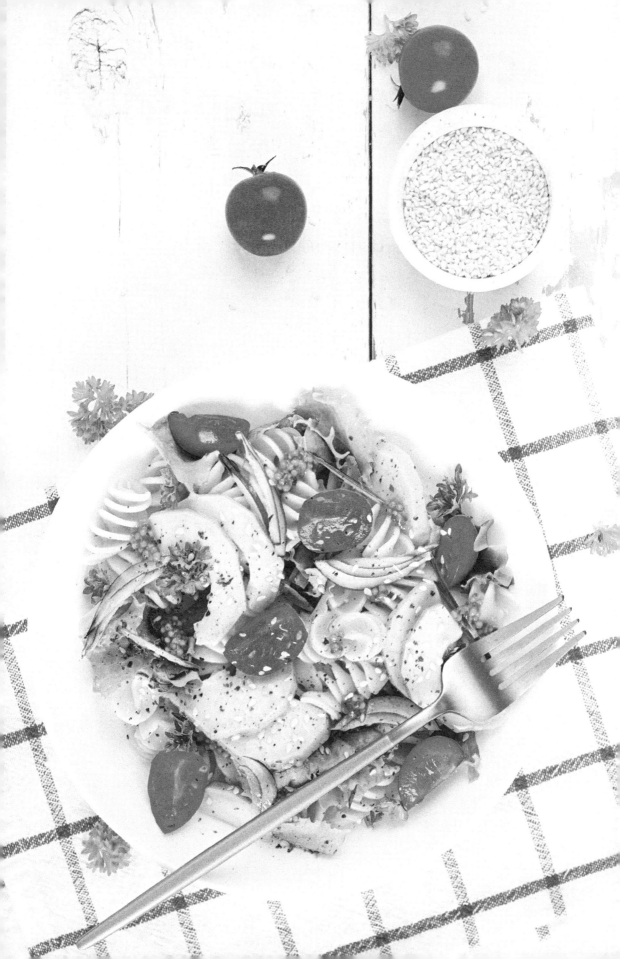

Table of Contents

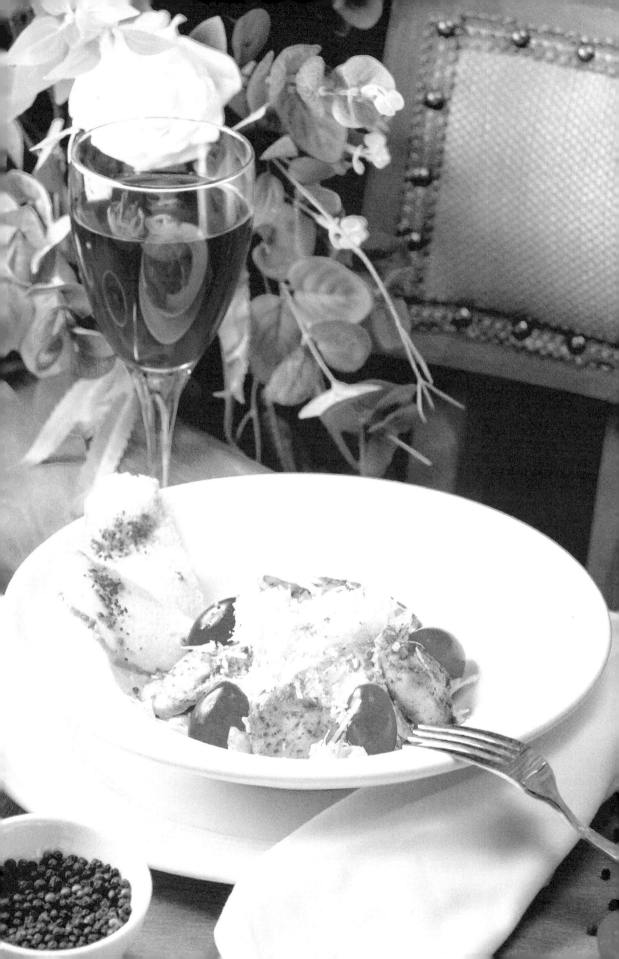

Introduction

Pregnancy brings with it a variety of changes. This is an incredibly special time in your life and a major milestone. Knowing that you are pregnant for the first time can elicit different emotions. From elation, happiness, and gratitude, to nervousness, anxiety, and worries, you experience it all. It's quite normal for women to feel extremely happy one moment and start panicking the next during their pregnancy. Unfortunately, this is also a stage where you'll be bombarded with unsolicited advice from all sources. Whether it is social media, information on Google, or advice given by well-meaning and seemingly all-knowing family members, friends, and even acquaintances. Everyone seems to have something to say about pregnancy and all things associated with it. When information starts coming at you from all directions, it might quickly become overwhelming. How do you know what works when so many people have so many opinions?

Before we get started, I believe congratulations are in order. Becoming a mother regardless of whether it's your first or the fourth time, will always be a wonderful experience. After all, bringing new life into this world is no small feat. The good news is that this book will act as your guide every step of the way. In this, you will discover guidance about the right nutrition not just during pregnancy but immediately after it as well.

The role played by nutrition cannot be overlooked. This is the cornerstone of health and there is no way around it. The information given in this book will help demystify prenatal nutrition. In this book, you will learn about the different nutrients your body requires during this period and the benefits associated with them.

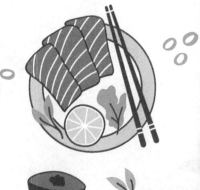

After this, you will learn about the different changes your body undergoes during each of the trimesters. You will also be introduced to fetal development during pregnancy. Once you know the importance of nutrition and the different nutrients to focus on, taking care of your health becomes easier. This book not only caters to the three trimesters of pregnancy but includes the fourth trimester too. Are you wondering what this is? It includes helpful information for new moms right after delivery.

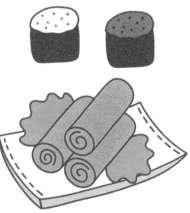

Having this book by your side will give you the required nutrition to efficiently wade through the pregnancy without compromising on nutrition. This is the only means to ensure you and the baby are moving along healthily. This book is filled with a variety of healthy, nutritious, and delicious recipes. All these recipes are quite simple to cook and can be whipped up within no time. You needn't spend hours together in the kitchen. Doing this might not be possible during pregnancy. If you are looking for simple and delicious recipes that cater to your body's changing nutritional requirements, then look no further. Simply find the recipes that strike your fancy, gather the needed ingredients, and follow the instructions. This coupled with the information given about prenatal nutrition will make things easy for you! So, dear soon-to-be-mama, it is time to get started!

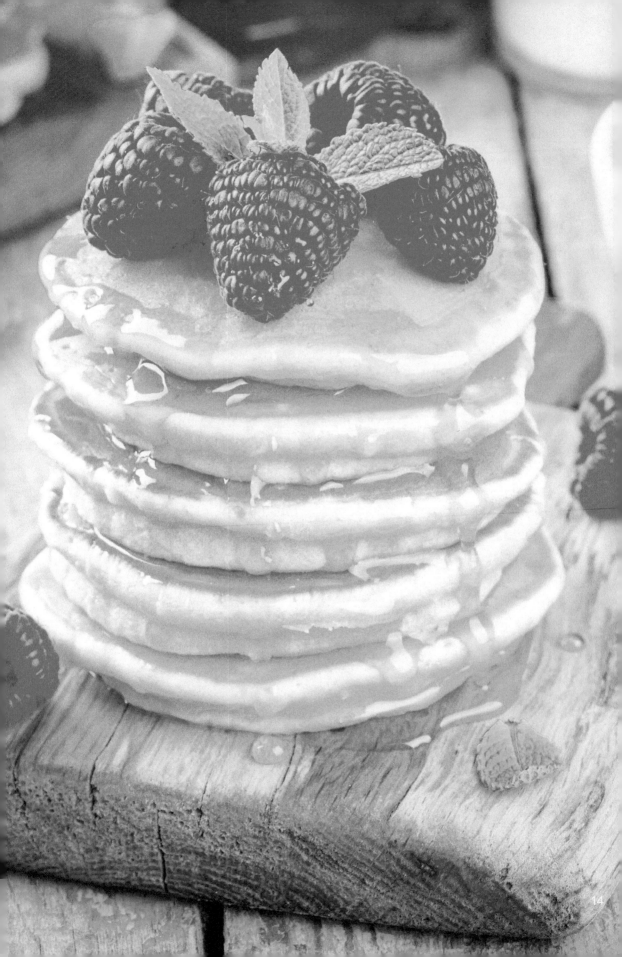

CHAPTER ONE

It Starts With Prenatal Nutrition

"The first wealth is health."
Emerson

A healthy diet is one of the essential pillars for your overall health and sense of well-being. The role of diet is even more important during pregnancy. The diet you follow can leave a lasting effect on your baby's health for the rest of their life. Eating well to support a healthy pregnancy isn't difficult once you know what you are supposed to and are not supposed to do. The foods you opt for shouldn't be of any potential danger to your baby and must contain the required nutrients needed for your health too. Apart from all this, they must taste good as well. You might have heard that you need to eat for two during pregnancy. This looks a lot different than the eating habits you've been used to so far. Well, you don't have to worry because all the information you require about nutrition as a first-time mother is given in this book.

One of the most common questions pregnant women ask is about all the foods that they are not supposed to eat. Unfortunately, many have heard of different lists of foods they must avoid during pregnancy. However, most are not even aware of the foods that they should be eating. There will certainly be some foods that must be avoided. Whether it is sushi or a rare steak, avoid them during your pregnancy. Apart from this, you need to focus on eating foods that offer the nutrients your body and the fetus in your womb require. Dear mama, it's no longer just about catering to your health. Instead, you now have the responsibility of taking care of your little one too.

An important thing to remember is to understand that eating healthily during pregnancy doesn't have to be complicated and it certainly doesn't have to be filled with trendy foods such as goji berries. Instead, you need to focus on a well-balanced approach that consists of nutrient-dense foods. Pregnancy-fueling nutrients such as healthy fats, protein, choline, and folate are needed. Contrary to all things you have heard so far remember there is no such thing as a single superfood for pregnancy. Instead, you need to consume a variety of foods. Even all those that are usually labeled unhealthy such as an occasional donut or a slice of cake, especially the ones fueled by pregnancy cravings are quite normal. You don't have to give up on all these foods for the sake of your health. Instead, it is about learning to eat what your body requires and then moving on to anything else.

Focus on the Building Blocks of Nutrition

Before you start learning about the different foods you can eat during your pregnancy, it's important to understand the basic building blocks of nutrition you need to focus on. The three primary things you need to remember are calories, macronutrients, and micronutrients.

Calories

We all keep using the word calories in regular conversations, but most don't know what it means. So, what are calories? A rudimentary explanation is that calories are a unit of energy present in the food you consume. Calories are the energy your body requires to function effectively and efficiently. That said, all calories are not the same. Some are healthy while others are not. For instance, calories are present in a bowl of salad as well as a bag of cookies. However, only one of them is healthy.

Understand that you will need to consume more calories than usual during pregnancy. After all, it requires extra energy to grow and support the development of a little human within your body. This energy requirement further increases if you are carrying multiples. During the first trimester, your energy requirement will stay the same as any other phase in life. However, this steadily increases as the pregnancy progresses. Even if you have to increase your calorie intake, understand that it needs to come from nutrient-dense foods. This means it's not about eating a bag of cookies and thinking you have hit your daily calorie requirement. Usually, the calorie requirement during the first trimester is around 1800. This increases to 2200 and 2400 calories per day during the second and third trimesters, respectively.

Macronutrients

As mentioned, calories are present in any food you eat. They come in the form of three macronutrients which are the building blocks of nutrition. These macronutrients are proteins, carbohydrates, and fats. They serve specific functions and play important roles in your body. Their roles are further amplified during pregnancy. Ensure that the diet you follow includes the healthy dose of the three macros unless your doctor says otherwise. You will learn more about the macronutrients later in this chapter, for now, let's get back to the basics of nutrition.

Micronutrients

All the other vitamins and minerals your body requires that are not included in the above-mentioned macros are known as micronutrients. As the name suggests, you only need them in small quantities. That said, they play an extremely important role in prenatal health. Here are some crucial nutrients you must focus on for a healthy pregnancy.

Calcium

The recommended dosage of calcium during pregnancy as well as lactation is 1000 mg per day. Taking a high dose of calcium and iron is not recommended since these nutrients compete for their absorption in the body. If you are using a supplement, ensure that it does not contain more than 500 mg of calcium at any given time. Calcium is needed for improving and supporting the baby's development of bones, muscles, nerves, and heart. Lack of sufficient calcium during pregnancy, especially in the third trimester, increases the risk of developing brittle bones and can result in osteoporosis in the mother.

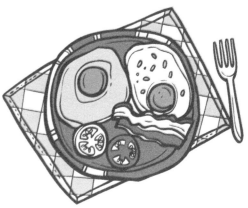

Dietary sources of calcium include dairy products such as milk, cheese, and yogurt. Dark green leafy vegetables along with legumes such as Brussels sprouts, mustard greens, and collards must be added to your diet. You can also consume foods that are fortified with calcium such as breakfast cereals and orange juice.

Choline

Choline is known as a brain-building nutrition and is needed for promoting cognitive functioning in the baby along with the development of their neural tube. The recommended dosage of choline during pregnancy is 450 mg per day and 550 mg per day during lactation. The best dietary sources of choline include peanuts, cruciferous vegetables, beef, chicken, fish, nuts, pork, and egg yolks.

Folate

Vitamin B9 is also referred to as folate. Consuming a sufficient amount of this vitamin is known to reduce the risk of birth defects in a baby, promote the production of DNA and helpful cells, and reduce the risk of cleft palate as well. It reduces the risk of the baby developing birth defects such as spina bifida that harm the baby's spinal cord. The synthetic form of this vitamin is known as folic acid, and it is converted into folate within the body. It is also believed that consuming sufficient folic acid reduces the chances of heart defects along with birth defects in the baby. The recommended dosage of folate is 400 mcg per day during pregnancy and around 500 mcg per day during lactation. The most common sources of folate include dark green leafy vegetables, citrus fruits, beetroot, nuts and seeds, berries, and avocados.

DHA

DHA stands for docosahexaenoic acid, and it is a type of omega-3 fatty acid. Don't worry about looking at the term fatty acids because these are helpful fats your body requires. These heart-healthy fatty acids are not just good for the mother's health but her baby's too. A little over 20 mg per day is needed during pregnancy and lactation. This essential nutrient is needed for the growth and development of the fetus and plays an important role in fetal neurodevelopment and promotes the growth of the brain, skeletal muscle, and eyes. The risk of preterm birth reduces when your body obtains sufficient DHA during pregnancy. The most common dietary source of DHA includes seafood that's low in mercury such as halibut, scallops, herring, anchovies, and salmon. Eggs, milk, and orange juice fortified with DHA can also be added to your diet.

Iron

Iron is a helpful mineral that's utilized by the body for producing a protein known as hemoglobin. This is responsible for transporting oxygen from the lungs to all cells in the body. During pregnancy, the requirement for iron increases significantly. This is needed to ensure sufficient red blood cells are produced which ensures the needed oxygen is transported to your growing baby. The recommended dosage of iron during pregnancy is 27 mg per day and 9 mg during lactation. The requirement for iron doesn't increase until the second trimester. However, if there is excess blood loss during labor, your iron intake needs to increase. The iron requirement also increases once your menstrual cycle sets in after childbirth. It is an essential nutrient because it supports the blood supply the growing baby requires. It also aids the healthy production of red blood cells while reducing the risk of anemia in the mother and baby. It encourages fetal brain development by delivering the required oxygen to the growing fetus. Dietary sources of iron include beef, sardine, chicken, eggs, white beans, spinach, dark chocolate, lentils, and cashews.

Vitamin A

Vitamin A plays an important role in regulating and strengthening immune functioning. It is needed for maintaining the immune health and functioning of the mother as well as her baby during pregnancy. This vitamin also promotes proper development of the baby's organs and skeleton and is needed for their eye health too. During pregnancy, you'll need around 770 mcg RAE (retinol activity equivalent). Higher doses aren't recommended and during lactation, the requirement increases to 1200mcg RAE. Milk is an excellent source of vitamin A your body requires. Any food that's naturally orange-colored such as carrots, sweet potatoes, apricots, cantaloupe, and pumpkins is also rich in a naturally occurring form of vitamin A known as beta carotene which is later converted to vitamin A within the body. Even dark leafy greens are a good source of this vitamin. Another form of vitamin A your body needs is retinol. Retinol is needed to maintain skin health and its common sources include cod liver oil, animal fats, beef liver, and naturally fatty fish.

Iodine

Iodine is an important nutrient, especially for the development of the baby's brain. Therefore, your iodine intake needs to increase during pregnancy. Excess iodine isn't good. So, ensure that you do not over-supplement this nutrient. If its level is too low, it reduces the thyroid levels. This, in turn, causes different complications during pregnancy such as preterm birth, and an increased risk of miscarriage, and can result in poor growth of the fetus as well. The recommended intake of iodine during pregnancy and lactation must be around 250 mcg per day. Any supplement of iodine must contain at least 150 mcg per day and no more. The ideal nutrient source of iodine is potassium during pregnancy. The most common sources of healthy iodine include iodized salt for cooking roasted, seaweed, and cod.

Vitamin D

Vitamin D is fat-soluble and plays a crucial role in pregnancy. It enables your body to absorb calcium. A deficiency in this during pregnancy increases the risk of the baby developing type-one diabetes and other health conditions later in life. During pregnancy and lactation, the recommended dosage of vitamin D is 600 IU per day. If you are using a vitamin D supplement, then opt for one which has vitamin D3 instead of vitamin D2. Vitamin D3 is easily absorbed by the body. It plays a crucial role in supporting the bone health and immune functioning of the developing fetus. It also reduces the risk of preterm birth. Another benefit is it reduces the risk of the baby developing cavities later in life. Certain types of seafood, fortified dairy products and cereals, milk, and egg yolk are excellent dietary sources of this essential vitamin.

Prenatal Vitamins

By now, you would have understood the crucial role played by different nutrients during pregnancy. Consuming a well-balanced diet ensures that your body and growing fetus have the required nutrients. However, using a supplement or prenatal vitamins is a good idea to bridge any nutritional gaps in the diet. It's highly unlikely to obtain the required amount of each nutrient every day through food. By using prenatal vitamins, this nutritional gap is covered. Usually, it is recommended that anyone trying to conceive must start taking prenatal vitamins at least three months before conception. Well, if this does not apply to you, it is never too late to start taking them.

The type of prenatal vitamins you need to take or that dosage varies depending on several factors such as the diet you are following, your existing health status, and your general lifestyle. For instance, the prenatal vitamin formulation a vegan requires will be quite different from someone who consumes animal foods regularly. It's always recommended to consult your doctor and obtain personalized supplementation advice. That said, there are some general guidelines you need to remember while selecting a supplement or prenatal vitamins.

The prenatal vitamins you opt for must include folic acid, vitamin D, calcium, vitamin C, thiamine, riboflavin, niacin, vitamin B12, vitamin E, zinc, iron, and iodine. The ideal dosage of these nutrients in the prenatal vitamins must be as follows.

- Folic acid–400 mcg
- Vitamin D–400 IU
- Calcium–200 to 300 mg
- Vitamin B12–6 mcg
- Vitamin C–70 mg
- Thiamine–3 mg
- Riboflavin–2 mg
- Niacin–20 mg
- Vitamin E–10 mg
- Iron–17 mg
- Zinc–15 mg
- Iodine–150 mcg

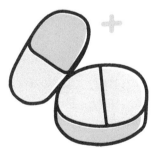

A vitamin D supplement will be needed if you aren't exposed to sufficient sunlight daily. Similarly, the B12 and zinc requirements of those following a predominantly plant-based diet such as vegan or vegetarian diets will be higher. An iron supplement is commonly prescribed during the second and third trimesters. While using an iron supplement, your intake of vitamin C must increase to promote better iron absorption. So, a vitamin C supplement will be prescribed if an iron supplement is needed. Some pregnant women benefit from using a probiotic supplement for maintaining healthy bowel movements, a B6 supplement to relieve nausea, and magnesium for alleviating cramps.

At times, the iron present in prenatal vitamins you take can result in constipation. That said, constipation can be easily managed if you increase the intake of fluids and dietary fiber. Apart from this, adding some physical activity to your daily routine is also recommended. That said, ensure that you consult your healthcare provider before exercising regularly. If these suggestions don't help, then don't hesitate to seek medical help.

NOTE: Do not make any dietary changes or add supplements without consulting your healthcare provider.

Foods to Eat

By now you are aware of the importance of a balanced diet during pregnancy. Now it is time to look at all the different foods you can enjoy while ensuring that you have a healthy pregnancy.

Whole Grains

One topic that the Internet is divided about is carbohydrates. This is a topic on which you should not obtain any information from the Internet or social media. There are plenty of self-proclaimed nutrition experts who believe carbohydrates in any form are nothing but pure evil. They are the ones that recommend the complete elimination of carbohydrates.

That said, it's important to understand that carbohydrates are one of the three macronutrients your body requires. They are an important source of energy and contain dietary fiber. Apart from it, they also contain essential vitamins, minerals, and antioxidants your body requires. So, cutting them all out of your diet is not a good idea.

Similarly, all carbohydrates are not the same. Some are healthy while others are not. An important group of carbohydrates that must be included in your pregnancy diet are whole grains. Due to different personal health reasons, some opt for a grain-free or a gluten-free diet. Some whole grains such as quinoa and corn are gluten-free and can still be consumed. Any grain that can be consumed in its entirety or whole form is known as whole grains. Some excellent examples of whole grains your body requires are corn, oats, wheat, sorghum, spelt, barley, corn, quinoa, rice, and rye.

Instead of refined grains such as white flour, white bread, white rice, and any other products made with them, replace them with whole grains. Whole grain flour, brown rice, and whole-grain bread are excellent alternatives for refined ones. Consuming sufficient whole grains offers essential dietary fiber. This is needed for regulating bowel movements and promoting satiety. Once the grains are processed or refined, the natural fiber in them is eliminated. This is one of the reasons why whole brown rice is much better than refined white rice.

Consuming antioxidants is needed, especially during pregnancy to tackle naturally occurring oxidative stress. Whole grains that were mentioned above are rich in natural antioxidants along with pregnancy-fueling nutrients such as iron, B complex vitamins, and magnesium. These are also slow-digesting when compared to refined carbohydrates. This, in turn, reduces the risk of any spikes in blood sugar levels. This is needed for stabilizing your energy levels and reducing the risk of developing diabetes. The nutrients present in whole grains are also good for a baby's growth and development. For instance, whole grains fortified with essential nutrients such as folic acid are important for the baby's development. Adding them to your diet is also incredibly simple. For instance, you can snack on homemade popcorn, replace white rice with quinoa, and enjoy sandwiches made with whole-grain bread instead of refined flour.

Healthy Fats

Fats are one of the most misunderstood and commonly demonized food groups. As with carbohydrates, all fats are not the same. It's important to remember that fats should not be eliminated from your diet instead, you must opt for the right type of fats. In the previous section, you were introduced to DHA, a type of omega-3 fatty acid that's good for fetal brain development. Foods that are usually rich in healthy dietary fats also contain essential fat-soluble vitamins such as vitamins A, E, D, and K. They are all needed for supporting a healthy pregnancy and optimizing the absorption of other essential nutrients. That said, consuming too much fat regardless of the type is unhealthy.

The fats that you must focus on are unsaturated and you need to stay away from trans fats. Avocado, plant-based oils, and nuts along with olive oil are excellent sources of healthy fats. All fats found in coffee creamers and prepackaged treats and snacks such as chips and cookies are unhealthy trans fats. If you notice the word trans-fat on any pre-packaged product, avoid it because they are extremely unhealthy.

A variety of helpful fat you must consume for a healthy pregnancy is an omega-3 fatty acid. It is commonly found in naturally fatty fish and seafood, but you can obtain it from foods that are fortified with it such as orange juice and milk. Consuming the required omega-3 fatty acids is known to support mental health and reduce the risk of the mother developing postpartum depression.

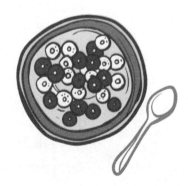

Proteins

Protein requirement increases during pregnancy. It is a building block for cells and muscles. Unsurprisingly, it is needed for promoting the baby's growth and development. The most common dietary sources of protein include meat, seafood, eggs, nuts, and eggs. The usual requirement of protein during pregnancy is around 60 grams per day. Ensure that most of the protein that you opt for is from lean sources such as meat without any fat, eggs, and seafood. Lean protein contains lower levels of saturated fat and is lower in calories too. This means, your pregnant body obtains the required dose of protein without increasing the calorie consumption. It, in turn, makes it easier to accommodate other food groups.

The dietary sources of lean protein are also rich in essential nutrients such as zinc, iron, and even vitamin B 12. Your body also requires certain essential amino acids from meat and other dietary sources. However, the intake of fatty meat must be in moderation. If you are following a plant-based diet such as a vegan or vegetarian lifestyle, you need to include healthy plant-based protein options such as lentils and peas. However, these are not rich in the essential amino acids your body requires. In such instances, opting for a dietary supplement is needed but ensure that you consult your healthcare provider before doing it.

Fruits and Veggies

An important dietary change that anyone can make regardless of their stage of life is increasing the consumption of healthy and wholesome fruits and vegetables. A simple rule you can follow is to eat the rainbow. It essentially means your diet must include a variety of fruits and vegetables of different colors. Incorporating fruits and veggies of different colors ensures that a variety of nutrients and essential vitamins and minerals your body requires are automatically obtained. They also offer a variety of benefits that cannot be replicated by any supplements or prenatal vitamins.

Another important reason why fruits and vegetables must be a part of your diet is they are a rich source of dietary fiber. A common side effect most women experience during pregnancy is constipation. Certain levels of hormones increase during pregnancy which causes relaxation of intestinal muscles. This, in turn, reduces the frequency of bowel movements or makes it difficult. Also, the added pressure of an expanding uterus can make you feel constipated. The best way to alleviate these symptoms is by consuming plenty of dietary fiber. Plant-based foods are the best source of dietary fiber you can get your hands on.

Seafood

The best source of essential fatty acids your body requires is seafood. They contain two helpful fatty acids known as DHA and EPA. Your body cannot produce these fatty acids and they cannot be obtained from plant-based foods. Consuming DHA and EPA is important for supporting eye and brain development in the fetus. It also reduces the risk of mothers developing postpartum depression. That said, there are some caveats involved when it comes to consuming fish and shellfish during pregnancy.

Seafood usually contains different toxic metals, especially mercury. Consuming too much mercury puts your baby at risk of developing certain health problems. Therefore, you need to consume seafood such that you obtain the required DHA and EPA along with other nutrients without increasing the consumption of harmful heavy metals. Certain seafood has less mercury than others. Large fish prey on small ones. Therefore, the level of mercury in the former is greater than in the latter. The most common fish you need to avoid due to high levels of mercury include swordfish, tuna, and marlin. Instead of them, you can opt for seafood that belongs to the lower rungs of the food chain such as shrimp, scallops, salmon, tilapia, and cod. Aim for two two-ounce servings each of seafood low in mercury. To ensure that you are obtaining sufficient DHA and EPA, you'll need to probably add a supplement upon the recommendation of your doctor.

Foods to Avoid

Until now, you were introduced to different foods you can enjoy during pregnancy. Now, let's look at some you must avoid or consume only in moderation for a healthy pregnancy. If you love coffee or are a sushi lover, giving up on your favorite foods can be quite a bummer. Fortunately, there are plenty of foods you can eat. Instead of focusing on all that you cannot eat, concentrate on the ones you can. By keeping an open mind, it becomes easier to see that pregnancy is by no means restrictive. Also, the different healthy and delicious recipes given in this book will ensure that you don't feel like you are missing out on tasty meals! Here are some foods that you need to avoid or minimize while pregnant.

Certain Types of Fish and Seafood

Avoid fish that is high in mercury such as marlin, tuna, swordfish, and shark. Not all fish and seafood are high in mercury, and you can always opt for low-mercury fish such as anchovies, salmon, and trout. They are also an excellent source of lean protein and healthy omega-3 fatty acids. Consuming at least 2 servings of low-mercury seafood is good for your health and that of your baby during the pregnancy.

This will be tougher for anyone who loves sushi. However, you need to stay away from undercooked or raw fish. Raw fish and shellfish can cause a variety of infections. Some might only affect you, but others can be passed on to the baby with serious consequences. So, stay away from raw fish and shellfish including sushi and other similar preparations during pregnancy.

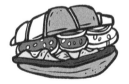

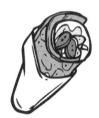

Processed, Raw, and Undercooked Meat

As with raw fish, you need to avoid undercooked meat too. Eating raw or undercooked meat increases the risk of contracting different bacteria or parasitic infections such as the ones caused by listeria, salmonella, and E. Coli. Such infections can become life-threatening for your little one. If you love your steak rare or medium-rare, you need to make a few changes. Ensure that all the meat you consume is fully cooked. Similarly, you need to stay away from processed meats such as cold cuts, deli meats, and hot dogs. The processing process coupled with storage leaves such foods exposed to a high risk of contamination.

Raw Eggs

Raw eggs are at risk of being contaminated by salmonella bacteria. Salmonella poisoning and infection can induce vomiting, severe stomach cramps, fever, and diarrhea. In some rare cases, this infection can result in premature or stillbirth due to excessive cramping of the uterus. Whether it is poached eggs, homemade ice cream, homemade mayonnaise, or even hollandaise sauce, avoid anything that has raw eggs in it. Ensure that you always consume eggs that are thoroughly cooked or opt for pasteurized eggs.

Unpasteurized Products

A variety of harmful bacteria such as salmonella and E.coli are present in unpasteurized dairy products such as raw milk and unpasteurized cheese and soft cheeses. This applies to unpasteurized juices as well. These infections can be tolerated by an adult but can be life-threatening for an unborn baby. The bacteria can either be naturally occurring or can be due to contamination during collection or the storage stages. Whatever the reason, it's better to opt for pasteurized products to minimize the risk of infections. Whether it is cheese, juice, or milk, opt for only pasteurized products.

Caffeine

If you love your daily cup of coffee comedy or any other caffeinated beverage, this is going to be a tricky change to make. It's better to limit caffeine throughout your pregnancy and breastfeeding stages. Yes, you need to limit it instead of avoiding it. Ensure that your caffeine intake is less than 200 mg per day. Whenever you consume any caffeinated beverage, the caffeine is first absorbed by your body and then it directly moves to the placenta. The enzyme needed to metabolize caffeine is absent in babies and their placentas. This can result in caffeine buildup which is harmful to fetal growth and health. High caffeine intake during pregnancy restricts fetal growth and increases the chances of the baby being underweight at birth. Low birth weight exposes your baby to an increased risk of chronic health problems later in life and can prove fatal in extreme cases. So, for the sake of your baby's health be extra mindful of the caffeine consumed.

Raw Sprouts

Sprouts are healthy and are a powerhouse of nutrients. Your idea of a healthy salad might include alfalfa or mung bean sprouts. However, you don't have to give up on sprouts altogether. Instead, understand that it's raw sprouts that are harmful because they can be contaminated with harmful bacteria. The humid 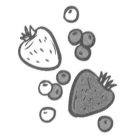 environment needed for sprouting becomes the perfect place for bacteria to grow and thrive. Getting rid of all traces of such bacteria is not possible even after thoroughly washing the sprouts. This is the reason why it is better to avoid raw sprouts altogether. However, you can consume them after they are cooked.

Alcohol

To reduce the risk of miscarriage and stillbirth, avoid alcohol during pregnancy. It needs to be further avoided after delivery if you plan to breastfeed. Even a small amount of alcohol consumed during pregnancy can impair your baby's brain development. It also increases the risk of fetal alcohol syndrome which can cause heart defects and other disabilities as well as deformities in the baby.

Junk Food

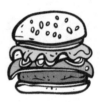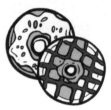

There is no time like the present to shift to a healthier diet. An even better reason to stay motivated while kicking the junk food habit is to consider the nutrition needed during pregnancy. Opting for nutrient-dense and wholesome foods is a better option any day. Your calorie intake will not increase dramatically during pregnancy. However, please ensure the calories you consume are from healthy and wholesome foods instead of unhealthy processed junk food. Most processed foods and beverages are rich in calories and harmful additives with little or no nutritional value whatsoever. The low-nutrient and high carb, sugar, and unhealthy fat junk food will not do you or your baby any favors. So, stay away from them!

Apart from all the different things mentioned until now, another thing you need to do is ensure that the produce you eat is thoroughly washed. The surface of unwashed fruit or vegetables can be contaminated with different types of bacteria as well as harmful pathogens. To minimize the risk of infection and the risk of infection spreading to your unborn baby it's important that you thoroughly wash the fruits or vegetables before consuming and. This is one habit that can stay up with you forever, and it's good for your health and that of your baby too.

Always Stay Hydrated

Staying hydrated is important. It's even more important during pregnancy because dehydration puts your baby at risk. Remember, your body is gradually growing and therefore, it requires more fluid to sustain the increased volume. Lack of fluids during pregnancy increases the risk of certain conditions such as low amniotic fluid and even premature labor. Regardless of your physical activity level, staying hydrated is needed. You'll need around 10 cups of fluid per day during the pregnancy. Ensure that you are drinking before you even feel thirsty. If needed, put a reminder on your phone or set alarms to ensure that you are drinking sufficient water.

A simple way to check whether you're hydrated or not is to see the color of your urine. If it is dark yellow or concentrated, it means you need more water. Some supplements can turn urine yellow regardless of your hydration status and in case of any doubt, don't hesitate to consult your healthcare provider immediately. If your body is not thoroughly hydrated, some common symptoms you can experience are headaches, dizziness, and tiredness. During the later stages of pregnancy, dehydration can trigger Braxton-Hicks contractions, also known as false labor.

Not just water, you can opt for infused water, coconut water, and fruit juices too. As much as possible, try to make fruit juices at home instead of relying on store-bought variants. The prepackaged juices also contain additives that aren't necessarily healthy.

Well-Balanced Portions

Pregnancy is an incredibly personal experience and it's not the same for everyone. This is one of the reasons why you need to consume healthy and well-balanced portions every day. This is not something you can overlook. After all, it's not just your health but your baby's health that is at stake too.

One thing you need to remember is that the portion sizes will not be the same for everyone. For instance, a woman who is physically active and is pregnant with multiples will require bigger portions and more calories than someone who leads a sedentary lifestyle and is pregnant with a single baby. Portion size is not the same as serving size. Serving size refers to the quantity which indicates the standard amount of food and the nutrition present in it such as an ounce or a cup. Here are some basic portion sizes you can remember to ensure that you are consuming well-balanced meals.

- Up to three ounces of poultry or meat. This portion size is similar to a deck of playing cards or the palm of your hand.
- Three ounces of seafood is equivalent to the size of a checkbook.
- One ounce of cheese is the same size as four dice put together.
- A medium potato or any other starchy vegetable will be equivalent to the size of a computer mouse.
- Two tablespoons of any nut butter such as peanut butter are equivalent to the size of a ping pong ball.
- If you are having any starch such as pasta, then you need a portion size that is equivalent to that of a tennis ball.

An ideal meal must not focus on a single category or food group. Instead, it needs to be an appropriate mixture of different food groups in required portions. For instance, instead of eating 2 or 3 big bowls of pasta for dinner, opt for a small bowl of pasta coupled with a healthy salad and some grilled protein of your choice such as chicken. Instead of a can of soda, opt for a glass of cold milk to deal with any of the pregnancy symptoms while ensuring your body gets its required dose of nutrition.

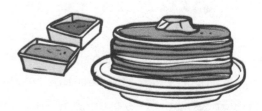

Celebrate the Journey

One thing you should not do at this stage is to start worrying about your weight. Most women gain a couple of extra pounds during pregnancy. This is the extra volume your body creates to support the growth of a baby on the inside. Don't be scared of it and instead embrace your pregnancy body. Focus on ensuring that you are healthy, and your body is strong enough to take care of your little one. The additional weight you put on is usually your baby's body mass, coupled with additional fluid and placenta.

Pregnancy is a wonderful experience, but it can be emotionally exhausting too. Going through your pregnancy for the first time is unlike anything else. Now is the time to be self-compassionate and focus on staying healthy and active. Every day will not be smooth sailing. There will be days when you don't feel like eating healthily or even getting up from the couch. It's okay, cut yourself some slack. Your body is trying to support and grow a little human on the inside. Do what feels right to you and don't hesitate to ask for support from others. Self-compassion must be a part of your daily routine and understand and recognize your body's cues. If you are worried about whether you are eating nutritious food or not, stop worrying because this book has got your back. In the following chapters, you will learn more about the different nutrients your body requires through all stages of pregnancy and after childbirth.

NOTE: Before you make any dietary changes, don't forget to consult your healthcare provider. This is even more important if you have any existing health conditions or problems.

Key Takeaways

- Nutrition plays a crucial role in maintaining not just your health but that of the growing fetus too.

- A healthy and well-balanced diet must be an ideal mixture of the three macronutrients and essential micronutrients.

- Important nutrients you need to focus on for a healthy pregnancy are carbohydrates, healthy fats, proteins, calcium, iron, vitamins A, B, C, D, and E, folate, calcium, iodine, and choline.

- Prenatal vitamins as prescribed by your healthcare provider are needed to bridge any nutritional gaps in your diet.

- The foods to stay away from during pregnancy include caffeine, alcohol, prepackaged and processed beverages, raw or undercooked meat and seafood, high-mercury seafood, processed meats, unpasteurized honey and dairy, and raw foods.

- Following a healthy diet helps tackle common pregnancy symptoms such as nausea, constipation, heartburn, and fatigue.

- Don't forget to cherish every moment of this journey because this is just the beginning of the greatest adventure of your life.

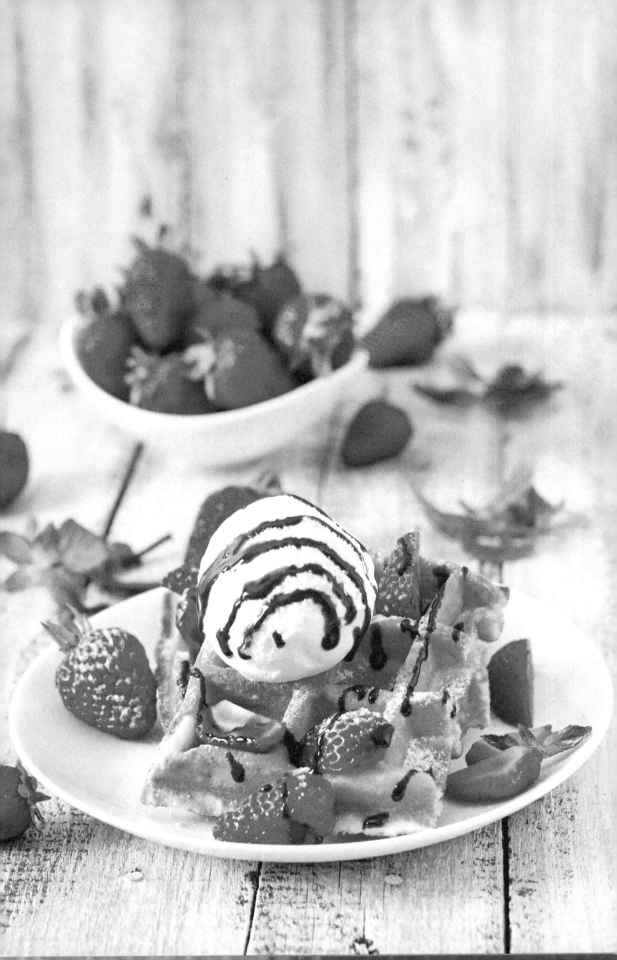

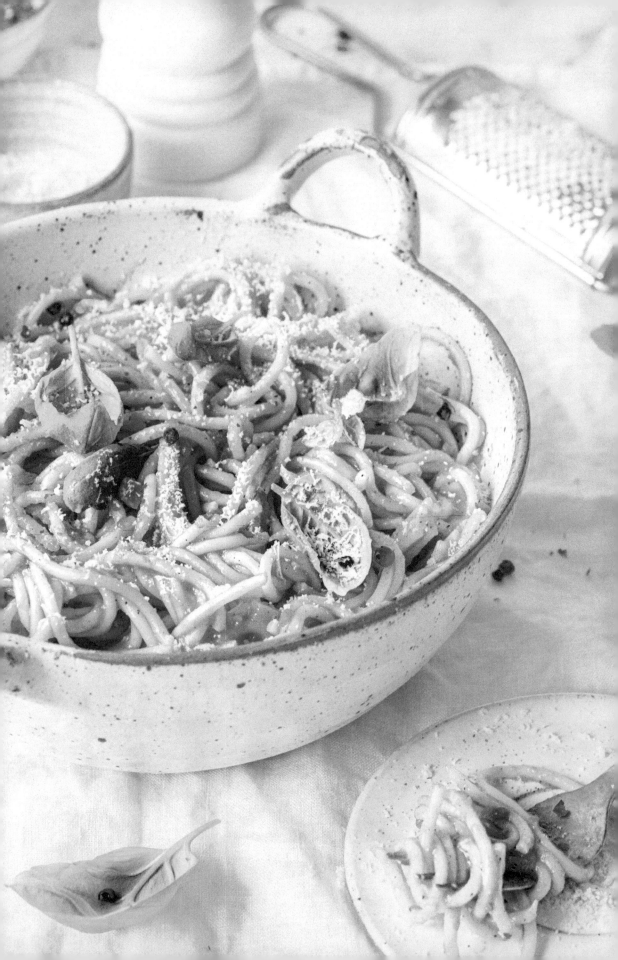

CHAPTER TWO

The First Trimester

_____

"To eat is a necessity, but to eat intelligently is an art."
La Rochefoucauld

Your pregnancy starts with the first trimester. Usually, the first three months are filled with excitement and the pregnancy glow that most experience. However, it also comes with its own set of unwelcome side effects such as morning sickness and nausea. Well, these are just temporary changes, and it essentially means your body is coping with the hormonal changes associated with pregnancy.

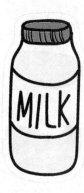

Certain hormonal changes take place during the first month to support the pregnancy. These hormones are responsible for the PMS-like symptoms most women experience during the first trimester such as mood swings, exhaustion, and nausea. Your calorie intake during the early stage of pregnancy needs to be around 1800 calories. This needs to increase if you are underweight to support a healthy pregnancy. The primary focus right now needs to be on the nutrients your baby requires for the development of the neural tube such as folic acid, vitamin B12, and choline.

These days, a variety of breakfast cereals and bread are fortified with folic acid. Green leafy vegetables and beetroots are excellent sources of folate which is a naturally occurring form of folic acid. You can reduce the risk of your baby developing certain birth defects by ensuring you consume sufficient choline. Different food sources rich in this nutrient were discussed in the previous chapter. The final nutrient you need to focus on is vitamin B 12. This coupled with choline and folic acid promotes and supports the fetus' neural tube development.

During this stage, your caffeine intake should be less than 200 mg per day. If you are used to drinking alcohol, smoking, or recreational use of drugs, now is the best time to stop it. Doing this is not just good for pregnancy but for your overall health in general too. The best foods for the first trimester are lean meat, yogurt, bananas, beans and lentils, kale and other leafy vegetables, and ginger tea.

During the first month, the sperm meets the egg. The embryo is then implanted into the uterus and this kickstarts the pregnancy journey. The major tell-tale sign of pregnancy is a missed period. Some might experience a little implantation bleeding, but this isn't the same as menstrual bleeding.

You'll start noticing some small changes in your body as you enter the second month of the first trimester. This is still an early stage of pregnancy, and you don't have to worry if you experience any PMS-like symptoms even now. Some might not experience any symptoms while others experience every possible symptom there is. The simplest way to combat them is by consuming fresh ginger and foods rich in vitamin B6. Dietary sources of vitamin B6 include chickpeas, nuts, and tofu. You should also focus on consuming sufficient choline, vitamin B 12, folic acid, and DHA. Apart from this, pay attention to your iodine intake too.

During the second month, your baby's neural tube is in the developing stage. Their face is also in the beginning stages of development along with the formation of essential organs such as lungs, kidneys, and liver. These will not be functional until the later stages of pregnancy, but their development starts now. The most common symptoms expectant mothers experience during the second month includes morning sickness, heartburn, mood swings, food cravings, and aversion to certain foods and smells. You will also notice your breast feels tender.

The third month of pregnancy brings us to the end of the first trimester. This is when you start getting accustomed to the idea of being a mother within a few months. Your baby is growing and developing by the end of this month and will be officially known as a fetus. If you are feeling fatigued, opt for nutrient-rich foods such as whole grains and fresh and fibrous vegetables and fruits. Your baby's bones start hardening and their fingernails start growing. To support this growth, you'll need to increase the consumption of calcium-rich foods. The fetus will start developing some exciting features such as teeth, muscles, bones, soft nails, and even intestines. You might experience food cravings, morning sickness and nausea, constipation, tiredness, and aversion to certain foods. Apart from it, your breasts will still feel tender, and you can experience lower back pain too.

Now, it's no longer just about you but your baby is also dependent on the food you eat. Therefore, you'll need to focus on consuming nutrient-dense foods to support the pregnancy. Also, opt for natural energy boosters to cater to your growing baby's requirements.

Tips to Deal With Morning Sickness and Nausea

If you are experiencing nausea, morning sickness, or an upset stomach, understand that this is just a temporary thing. These are symptoms associated with the first three months of pregnancy and here are some tips you can use to deal with them.

Instead of trying to eat three big meals every day opt for small meals. Ensure that you do not go for too long without eating because this can worsen the nausea you experience.

To ease any stomach discomfort and reduce digestive troubles avoid foods that are rich in unhealthy fats and stay away from spicy food too.

To deal with an upset stomach, opt for foods that have a soft texture and try to include plenty of fluids in your diet for a while. For instance, tolerating a healthy smoothie is easier than eating a large meal.

Keep a couple of easy-to-eat dry snacks handy to deal with nausea. Whether it's a handful of nuts, Graham crackers, or even pretzels, select some snacks you like and keep them with you at all times.

Another remedy to tackle morning sickness and nausea is to sip on a cup of freshly brewed ginger tea.

Key Takeaways

- The first trimester kickstarts the pregnancy journey.

- Essential nutrients that you need to focus on during this stage are folic acid, protein, iron, calcium, DHA, potassium, and vitamin C.

- The ideal calorie requirement during this stage is around 1800 calories per day and a little more if you are underweight.

- Now is also the time you can start taking prenatal vitamins as per your doctor's advice.

- The most common side effects experienced during the first trimester include constipation, fatigue, lower back pain, aversion to certain foods and smells, morning sickness, and tender breasts.

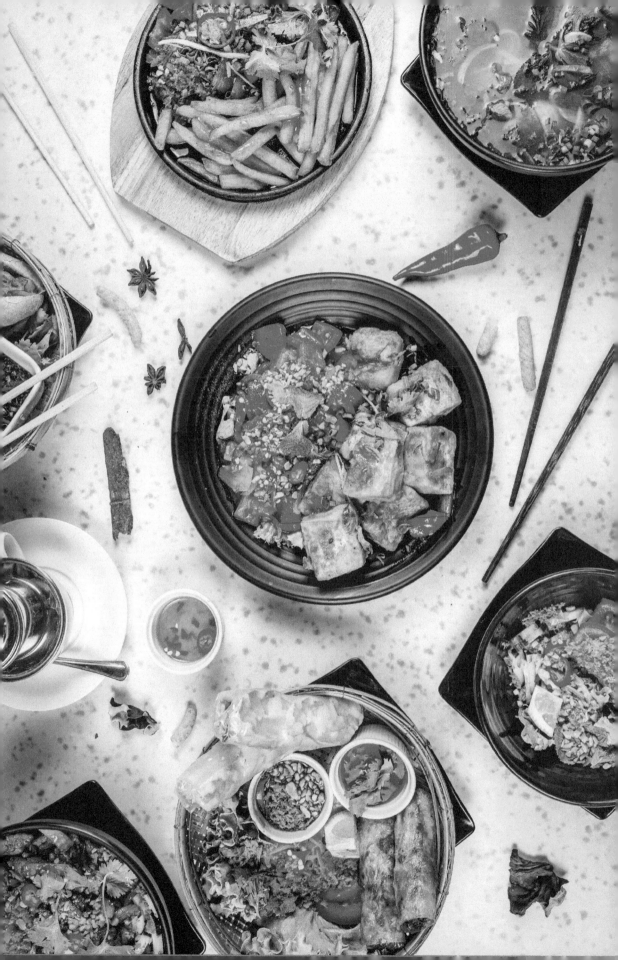

CHAPTER THREE

The Second Trimester

*"Our body is the only one we've been given, so
we need to maintain it; we need to give
it the best nutrition."*
Trudie Styler

Welcome to your second trimester! During these three months, fetal development moves ahead in full steam and some of the unwelcome pregnancy symptoms you experienced in the previous trimester subside. This is also the right time to start investing in comfortable maternity clothing because your body is going to change drastically. Eating during this trimester is relatively easier than the previous one because morning sickness and nausea along with tiredness you experienced will slowly go away. You'll feel quite good during the second trimester and make the most of the time available to consume nutrient-dense meals. Dear mama, it is time to enjoy the second trimester!

It's not just your body that will change, even your fetus is going to change quite a bit during the second trimester. By consuming the right foods, you can aid this natural development and relieve some of the unwanted side effects of pregnancy such as constipation. Focusing on dairy products is needed during this stage. A simple reason is that cold milk helps alleviate the heartburn and acidity you might experience. Similarly, calcium is needed for the development of your baby's bones and teeth. If you are not obtaining sufficient calcium during this stage, your body will prioritize the baby's growth and development. It means you will not have any calcium left for meeting your body's requirements because whatever is available will be redirected to the growing baby. Therefore, concentrate on consuming calcium-rich foods and opt for a supplement if your doctor recommends it.

Constipation is quite common during the second trimester and the best way to alleviate it is by consuming plenty of foods rich in dietary fiber. Whether it is whole grains, fruits with their skin, or cruciferous vegetables, go ahead and do it. You should also drink plenty of water to keep dehydration at bay and make it easier to move your bowels.

Dear mama, eggs and peanut butter are your best friends during this stage provided you aren't allergic to them. What more? The nutrients present in them promote your baby's brain development too. Another important nutrient you need to focus on for promoting your baby's born growth is magnesium. An excellent dietary source of magnesium is sweet potatoes. Also, increase your consumption of foods rich in iodine. This will have a positive role on your baby's brain health throughout its lifetime.

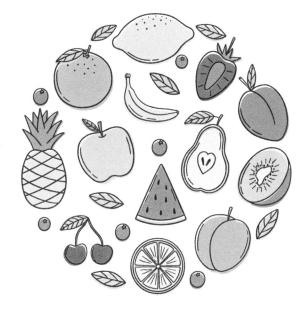

You can experience headaches during the second trimester for different reasons ranging from the food you consume to hormonal changes. Limiting the salt in your diet can help to a certain extent. You should also eat enough and stay hydrated to reduce headaches.

Usually, during the fourth month, the fetus can hear sounds, and its kidneys start functioning. Their heartbeat can also be heard through a doppler. Their teeth and bones become stronger while their eyes, eyebrows, eyelids, nails, and hair start forming. You can experience sleeping difficulties and constipation along with heartburn during the stage.

As you reach the fifth month you have hit the halfway point. During this month, your baby starts moving around and it might feel as if they are doing gymnastics in the womb. Feeling your baby kick for the first time is extremely exciting and a precious experience. They start to hear and now is a good time to start having conversations with your unborn baby. During this month, your primary focus must be to increase your intake of antioxidants. They not only reduce oxidative stress but help support your health during the rest of the pregnancy too. Food sources that are rich in natural antioxidants include all types of berries, squash, walnuts, black beans, and avocados. You will still need to focus on consuming a calcium-rich diet to support your baby's skeletal growth and formation and protect your bone health. When it comes to choosing dairy products, ensure that you always opt for pasteurized ones and stay away from all unpasteurized foods. As with the previous month, you need to increase your magnesium intake especially if you start experiencing any cramps. Another symptom you might need to deal with is heartburn. Having a glass of cold milk is a common remedy to reduce heartburn. Other simple suggestions include avoiding food that is spicy or acidic.

As you enter the sixth month of your pregnancy, you'll start feeling more than gentle kicks. Now is the time when you'll have a full-blown baby bump. Mama, don't forget to take some pictures to create beautiful memories for yourself. At this stage of pregnancy, your iron requirements will increase to support the higher volume of blood needed for the growing body inside your own. Consuming foods that are rich in iron such as spinach and beef help supplement this need. Similarly, you might also be recommended an iron supplement. One of the most common side effects of using an iron supplement is constipation. By staying hydrated and increasing your consumption of probiotic-rich foods and fibrous foods, you can tackle it. Another side effect is bloating. If you feel bloated most of the time, adding potassium-rich foods to your diet such as bananas, avocados, pistachios, and kiwis is helpful. Staying hydrated also reduces the risk of bloating.

If you are used to consuming any caffeine, now is the time to kick this habit, for a few months at least. Consumption of caffeine can affect iron absorption. Since iron is extremely important at this stage, avoiding caffeine is a good idea. You should also consume plenty of DHA-rich foods to promote your baby's brain development and growth. Apart from this, you'll need calcium and protein too.

At the sixth month mark, your baby's eyelids start parting and they can open their eyes. Their lungs are developed but are not yet functioning by themselves. They start developing sucking reflexes as well. Their vital organs are in the developing stage and are preparing themselves for surviving in the outside world once delivered. Apart from heartburn, bloating, and sleeplessness, prepare yourself for fuzzy memory as well. This is known as the pregnancy brain. The different hormonal changes that are going on in your body right now result in this condition. Remember this is just a temporary thing and it too shall pass. It's nothing to get worried about. Instead, focus on enjoying your pregnancy. You might notice that your ankles start to swell and stretch marks start appearing on your thighs and belly. As your body is accommodating the growing baby, it increases the pressure on the bladder. Therefore, be prepared for frequent trips to the loo to relieve yourself.

Some common foods that you can enjoy during the second trimester include milk, sweet potatoes, eggs, apples, peanut butter, whole grains, avocados, berries, cheese, squash, black beans, leafy greens, chicken, chocolate, watermelon, yogurt, salmon, almonds, and citrus fruits.

Key Takeaways

- Your baby's growth during the second trimester is quite prominent and quick. Physical changes will be noticed in your body too.

- The most common side effects of the second trimester you need to prepare yourself for include swollen ankles, the appearance of stretch marks, frequent urination, bloating, constipation, heartburn, and the pregnancy brain.

- Consuming a nutrient-dense diet and staying hydrated reduces these side effects while ensuring you and your baby get optimal nutrition.

- Apart from any doctor-prescribed prenatal multivitamins, the diet you follow must cater to your vitamin and mineral requirements too.

- Choosing foods containing omega-3 fatty acids, iodine, magnesium, folate, protein, iron, and vitamin C is helpful.

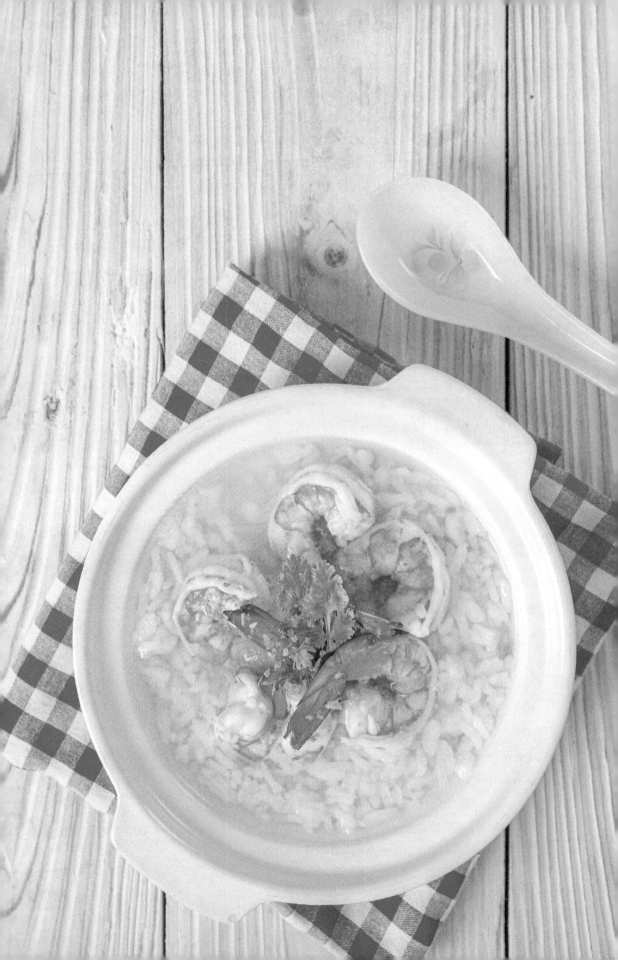

CHAPTER FOUR

The Third Trimester

"Of all the rights of women, the greatest is to be a mother."
Lin Yutang

You have entered the home stretch of your pregnancy and will be holding your little bundle of joy within a few months. Now your belly is bigger than ever before, your appetite will also increase drastically. While the preparations for your baby's arrival are in full swing don't forget about your nutrition and health too. You're almost there and as with the previous trimesters, keep consuming a healthy and well-balanced diet. Ensure that you are consuming a variety of foods to obtain the different nutrients you and your baby require.

Some general guidelines for your daily intake during the third trimester are as follows:

- Ensure that you are consuming 2-3 servings of lean protein or up to 75 grams of protein
- At least 3 servings of whole grains of your choice
- Around 4- 5 servings of nutrient-dense vegetables and fruits
- 4 servings of calcium-rich foods such as almonds, tofu, and dairy
- A minimum of one serving of healthy fats such as nuts, avocados, and seafood

During the third trimester, your baby's growth is accelerated. They start developing neural networks and brain tissue starts storing fat and working on their breathing. Their muscles and lungs start to mature, and their fingernails and toenails are developing too. All their major organs start functioning on their own except the lungs while their bones start hardening. Your baby's body is accumulating fat and is getting ready for life outside the womb. Towards the end of the third trimester, the baby usually assumes a head-down position also known as the breech position. This enables them to pass through the birth canal. So, now is the time to discuss your final birth plan with your doctor.

As your baby is growing and developing, you will also experience a recurrence of some of the symptoms you dealt with in the previous trimesters. Whether it is insomnia, frequent urination, constipation, or heartburn, prepare yourself for them. Remember, mama, you are in the last stretch, and now is the time to prepare yourself to welcome your bundle of joy into this world.

With all the different things happening within your body, the food choices you make are now more important than ever. The nutrients you require must be from low-fat pasteurized dairy, healthy fats and oils, fruits and vegetables, lean protein, and whole grains. A combination of all these different food groups ensures your body gets the required vitamins, minerals, and nutrients daily. The most important nutrients you need to focus on during the third trimester are vitamin A, vitamin C, vitamin B6, vitamin B 12, calcium, choline, iron, folate or folic acid, manganese, omega-3 fatty acids, protein, healthy fats, and oils, and whole grains.

Key Takeaways

- ✔ The third trimester marks the last leg of your pregnancy.

- ✔ While preparing for the arrival of your little one, don't forget to eat nutrient-dense foods and keep taking your prenatal multivitamin.

- ✔ Ensure that you are consuming plenty of fruits and vegetables daily along with whole grains and low-mercury seafood at least twice a week. Also, stay hydrated.

- ✔ Some of the symptoms you experienced during the first and second trimesters can reappear.

- ✔ Ensure that you are consuming foods rich in iron, vitamin C, manganese, omega-3 fatty acids, niacin, B-complex vitamins, protein, and calcium.

- During the third trimester, most of your baby's vital organs are fully functioning except their lungs. Their bones are hardening, and their body keeps growing and accumulating fat. In a way, your baby is preparing for its arrival into the world.

- The most common symptoms you need to prepare yourself for include Braxton-Hicks contractions, varicose veins, heartburn, pelvic pain, fatigue, constipation, and shortness of breath.

- Discuss your birthing plan with the doctor and keep a hospital bag packed for when the time arrives.

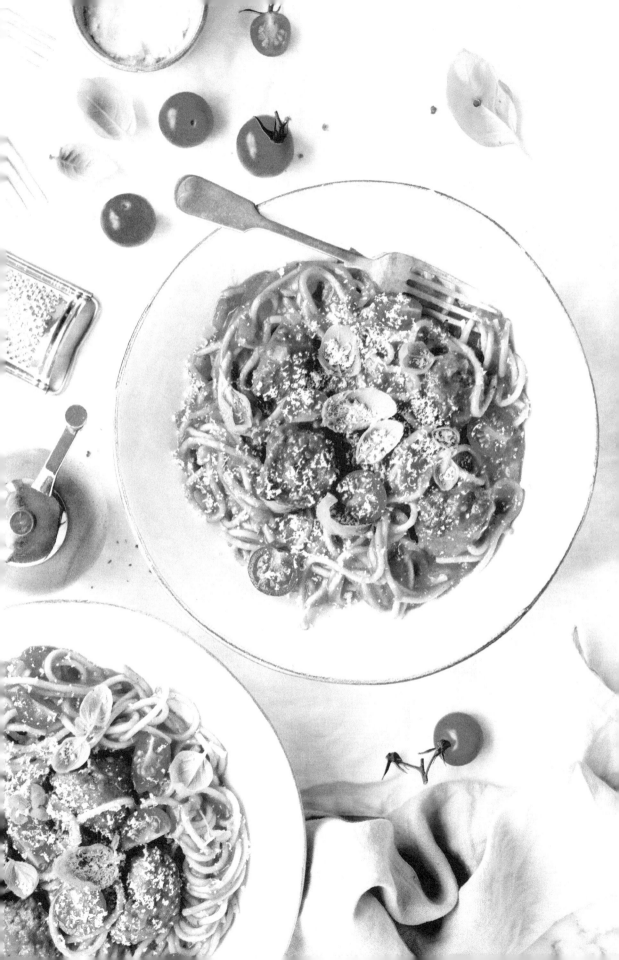

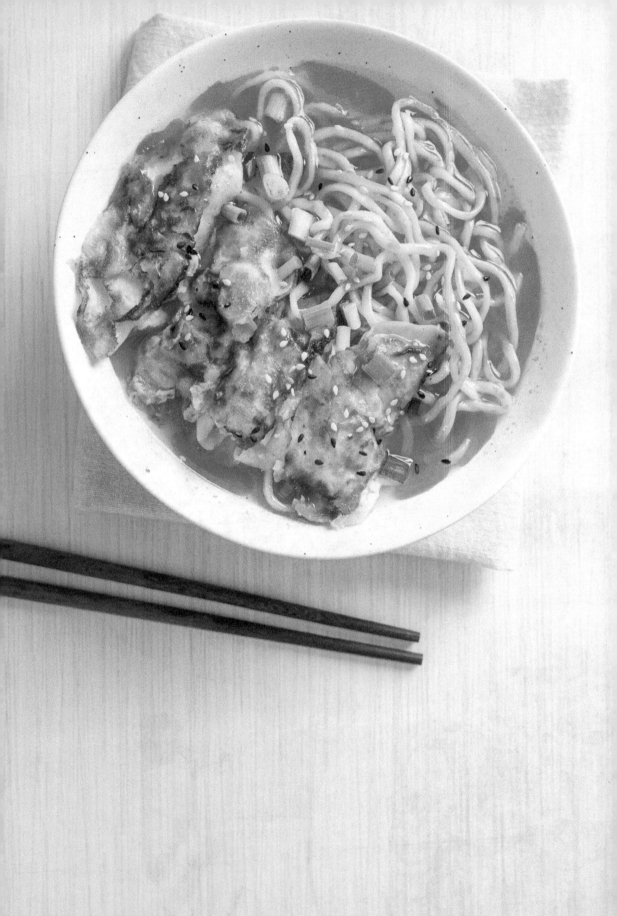

CHAPTER FIVE

The Fourth Trimester

"A grand adventure is about to begin."
Winnie the Pooh

You will receive nutrition information from a million sources when you're pregnant. You'll also be given unsolicited advice about the things you should be eating and not eating, and everything that you should and should not be doing. However, once your baby has arrived and you are healing from childbirth, this advice starts becoming leaner, especially from healthcare providers. This is the time when you should not only focus on your newborn but yourself too. As difficult as it can be to take time for yourself and focus on your healing, you should do it. After all, if you are not at your 100%, you cannot take care of your little one.

In this chapter, you will learn about all that you should be eating to support your healing after childbirth. Regardless of whether it's a C-section or a vaginal delivery, support yourself through your diet. Your dietary requirements further change if you are breastfeeding.

Heal Yourself

Welcoming a child into this world is a significant milestone. Giving birth is not an easy feat, regardless of whether it was a vaginal delivery or a C-section. You might have also exhausted yourself during labor. Apart from this, there's also blood loss and electrolyte loss during delivery. You can improve all these things by focusing on the right nutrition. Some also experience vaginal tearing or require additional surgeries after delivery. In such instances, focusing on the right food promotes healthy skin repair and makes a positive contribution toward your recovery. The most important nutrients you must focus on for postpartum healing are iron, protein, amino acids, micronutrients, and dietary fiber.

Experiencing blood loss during childbirth is common. Therefore, you must focus on rebuilding your blood count by increasing your intake of iron. Unless it's recommended by your doctor, opting for iron supplements is not recommended because it can result in constipation. Instead, you need to focus on consuming foods that are rich in iron such as legumes, leafy green vegetables, low-mercury seafood, beef, and chicken. Whenever you are consuming iron-rich foods, increase the intake of vitamin C to promote maximum absorption. So, some common foods that you can opt for are citrus fruits such as strawberries and oranges. Apart from those, cereals and oats that are fortified with iron also make for a convenient option.

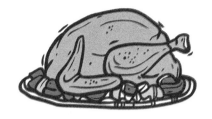

During pregnancy, your body will undergo significant and dramatic changes. Remember your body not just carried a new life within itself but supported its growth and development too. This means, your skin will stretch and change. Regardless of the type of delivery, healing takes plenty of time. During this stage, focusing on certain amino acids is needed because they support healthy skin. Proline and glycine are two crucial amino acids that are needed during your fourth trimester. Ideal food sources for these amino acids include poultry with skin, bone broth, and legumes. You can also opt for collagen peptides for supporting your skin health. However, ensure that your healthcare provider is on board with this idea.

Increase your protein intake because it helps rebuild and regrow the cells your body requires. Excellent dietary sources for protein include tofu, animal-based foods, and eggs. Apart from this, you also need a variety of micronutrients for improving and supporting skin health during the postpartum period such as zinc and vitamin C.

After childbirth, bowel movements can become quite challenging. To ensure that you stay ahead of constipation and support good bowel movements, it's important to increase your fiber consumption. Apart from dietary fiber, you should also drink plenty of water. The recommended consumption of fiber per day must be around 25-35 grams. Ideal dietary sources of fiber include fruit with skin, whole grains, vegetables, and certain seeds such as chia or flax seeds.

Nutrition Needs and Nursing

How you decide to nurse your baby is a personal choice. You can opt for formula feeding, breastfeeding, or a combination of two. As mentioned, your nutritional needs will change if you decide to breastfeed. Breastfeeding offers a variety of long-lasting benefits when it comes to your baby. However, certain nutrients present in breast milk are dependent on the diet you consume. Therefore, focusing on your nutrition is related to your baby's health if you decide to nurse them. Continuing with a prenatal vitamin is recommended for most lactating mothers. Even if you aren't breastfeeding, your diet must include the different nutrients discussed in this section.

One thing you need to do is stop obsessing about the calories consumed after childbirth. Now is the time to heal and recover from the rollercoaster ride your body underwent during the last nine months. Thanks to the online world filled with picture-perfect celebrities flaunting their bikini-ready bodies a few weeks after childbirth can create unrealistic expectations. A simple thing you need to understand is that your body has undergone a significant change. These changes occurred during pregnancy and didn't occur overnight. Even those extra pounds were not put on within a day or two. So, expecting to shed pregnancy weight and going back to your pre-pregnancy body cannot be an overnight process. Dear mama, cut yourself some slack. Not only is it too unsafe but is extremely unhealthy to severely cut down on your calorie intake immediately after childbirth. It is equally harmful to start exercising intensively during this period. If you have any doubts or worries about postpartum weight loss and want to become fit or lose weight, consult your healthcare provider. For now, the focus must be on getting stronger and healing your body and mind. While breastfeeding, you will need to consume an additional 400-500 calories per day.

While breastfeeding, your overall protein intake should also increase. You will need around 65 grams of protein per day. Therefore, you must opt for foods that are rich in protein, especially amino acids known as glycine. This promotes healing. Any food item that incorporates animal connective tissues such as bone broth or poultry with skin is helpful. Ensure that you have a couple of protein-rich snacks handy to cater to this need. A simple yet efficient means of obtaining your daily protein include hard-boiled eggs, some nut butter, and slices of fresh fruit. This is not only a quick snack but is easy to prepare too. With a little planning and preparation, taking care of your nutritional needs during the fourth trimester becomes easy.

Your intake of choline must also increase if you are breastfeeding. This is a vital nutrient in terms of the baby's brain development. Choline is transferred to your baby via breast milk. You'll need around 550 mg of choline per day during this period. Eggs are an excellent source of this vital nutrient. Since there are only so many egg yolks anyone can eat it is better to opt for a choline supplement. Ensure that you consult your healthcare provider before doing this. Cauliflower, animal liver, and peanuts are also other excellent food sources of choline.

In the previous chapters, you were introduced to an omega-3 fatty acid known as DHA which is needed for the baby's brain and vision development. A breastfeeding mother needs around 200-300 mg of this omega-3 fatty acid per day. It's not just good for the baby's health but your health too. It's needed for improving cognitive functioning and reducing the risk of any other mood-related disorders such as postpartum depression. Ideal food sources of this essential fatty acid are seafood. Ensure that you are consuming around two servings of low-mercury seafood such as shrimp, cod, trout, or salmon to obtain your required dose of DHA. If you are using any prenatal vitamins, then it will help hit the daily DHA requirement.

Selenium is an important antioxidant that promotes the metabolism of the thyroid hormone and supports immune functioning. Depending on your level of intake, its presence in breast milk is regulated. If you are consuming around two servings of low-mercury seafood, then you will obtain the needed selenium. If not, you will need to look for alternative sources. This is a nutrient that is not usually included in prenatal vitamins. An excellent source of selenium is Brazil nuts. So, add them to your daily diet!

Iodine is a vital nutrient. It plays a significant role in the development of your baby's brain as well as thyroid function. Apart from this, it is also important for you because it reduces the chances of any postpartum dysfunction of the thyroid and supports breast health. The requirement for iodine is higher in lactating women when compared to that during pregnancy. The simplest way to incorporate iodine into your diet is by using iodized salt. Apart from this common seafood, eggs, dairy products, and seaweed are also excellent sources of iodine.

The risk of a common health concern known as rickets can be reduced if you obtain sufficient vitamin D. A breastfeeding baby requires vitamin D supplementation of around 400 IU per day. Dear mama, you are not off the hook yet. Even you need sufficient vitamin D to promote your overall health and well-being along with your newborn's health. Depending on how much vitamin D you are obtaining, your baby's supplementation will vary. This is one thing that you need to consult your healthcare provider for before even getting started. Spending some time outdoors in the warm sunlight also does the trick. However, it's only during the early hours of the day when the sunlight is helpful.

Your baby's development is regulated to a certain degree by vitamin A. Your baby's ability to obtain this key nutrient is influenced by your intake. Vitamin A is needed for promoting the growth and development of your baby's immune system. Colostrum or the first breast milk that your baby has is an excellent source of this vitamin. It's also a 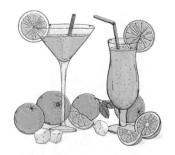 reason why it has a yellow tinge to it. The natural form of the vitamin is known as beta carotene and all foods that are naturally orange in color are excellent sources of it. While you are lactating, opt for foods rich in this nutrient.

There's a little reduction in your overall bone mass while breastfeeding. If your diet doesn't have sufficient calcium in it, then your infant's calcium requirement is obtained from your bones. To ensure this doesn't happen, you'll need to consume foods that are rich in calcium and vitamin C. Vitamin C promotes optimal absorption of calcium. Lactating mothers require up to 1000 mg of calcium per day to protect their bone health. As mentioned, ensure that you do not take a calcium supplement along with an iron supplement because these two minerals compete with each other for better absorption within the body.

Finally, do not forget about the importance of staying hydrated. Drinking more water doesn't mean your body can produce more breast milk. However, it's needed for your overall health and healing. Your body requires plenty of water to produce breast milk. Unless you replenish it, you cannot stay energized and healthy. Breastfeeding is tiring and if you don't have sufficient water and electrolytes, your energy levels will reduce.

What to Expect?

Now that your baby is out of your womb and is in the real world, it is all about them getting adjusted to it. Imagine how you would feel if you were plucked out of a dark, cozy, warm, and quiet environment and thrust into the world we know which is filled with different and strange smells, lights, and noises? Your baby can be cranky and will require plenty of love and attention at this stage. It's time for bonding with your child and nurturing them.

As important as it is to take care of your child, do not forget about yourself. There will be different changes you undergo as well during this period.

The first three months after childbirth are crucial because this is the time for self-care. As challenging as it sounds, self-care must be your priority too. You need to focus on healing your body and mind and consuming a healthy and well-rounded diet. Apart from this, you will also need plenty of rest to recuperate.

Key Takeaways

✓ The fourth trimester refers to the three months following childbirth. These are crucial not just for your newborn but for your health too.

✓ The primary focus should be on tending to your newborn's needs while healing your body and mind.

✓ Some essential nutrients you need to focus on at this stage or iron, protein, micronutrients, dietary fiber, and amino acids.

✓ Your nutrition needs will increase if you are breastfeeding.

✓ Instead of counting calories, focus on consuming protein, choline, omega-3 fatty acids, selenium, vitamins C, D, E, and B, and iodine-rich foods. Increase your consumption of calcium too.

✓ It takes a village to raise a child but don't forget about yourself in this process.

✓ Ask for the help that's needed, stock up on breastfeeding supplies, keep a postpartum care kit handy, and learn to say no. With a little care and consideration, you can be an excellent mother to your baby without ignoring your health.

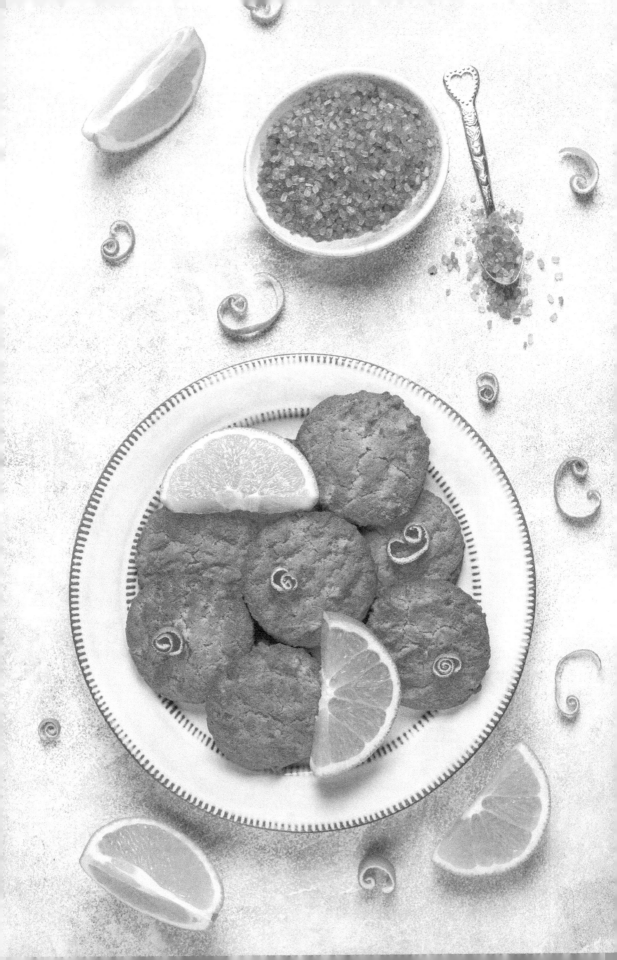

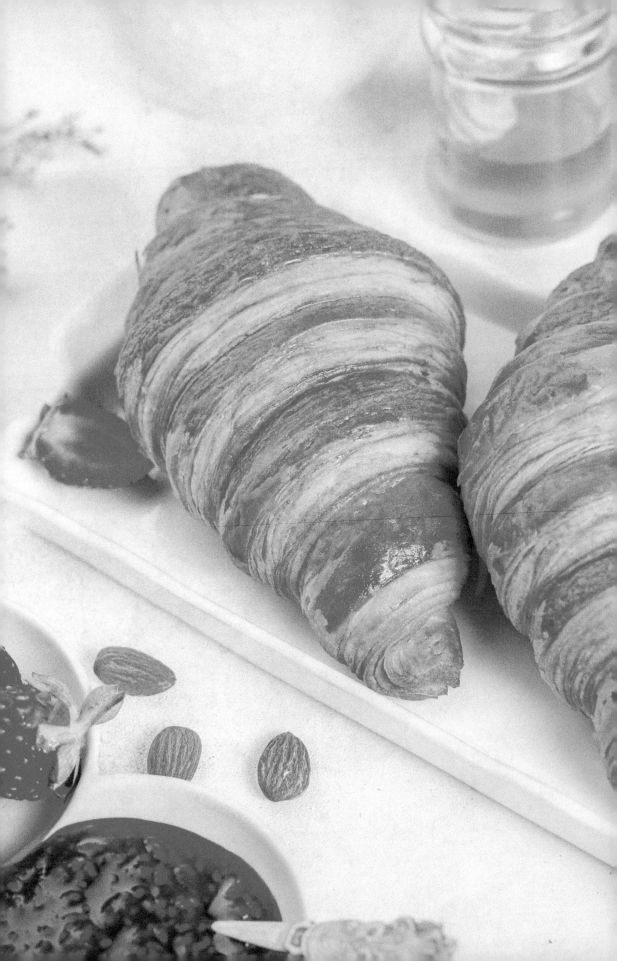

CHAPTER SIX

Eat Your Way Through Pregnancy

"Your diet is a bank account. Good food choices are good investments."
Bethenny Frankel

Some parts of the pregnancy are truly magical but there are some which are not so great and can become quickly overwhelming. Some do not experience any of the pesky pregnancy symptoms discussed in the earlier chapters. On the other hand, some experience every possible symptom under the sun. If you don't experience any of the pesky pregnancy symptoms it doesn't mean that something is wrong with you or that your pregnancy isn't normal. Understand that the human body is different, and we are all unique. Pregnancy is a highly personalized experience. The good news is that you have some control over how you feel. In this chapter, you will be introduced to different nutrition tips and suggestions that can be used for dealing with pregnancy symptoms along with dietary mistakes to avoid.

Nutrition and Pesky Pregnancy Symptoms

By now, you would have realized the important role of nutrition during pregnancy. Not just pregnancy, nutrition is important, period. This is one aspect of your life that you cannot overlook or compromise on because it's a fundamental pillar for your overall well-being. The most common pregnancy symptoms that are rather pesky to deal with include nausea and aversion to certain types of food, heartburn, constipation, and tiredness. A few healthy food choices here and there and some conscious effort will help reduce their intensity.

Morning Sickness

One of the most common pregnancy symptoms women experience, especially during the first trimester is nausea. At times, you can experience it during the second trimester as well. Food aversion is an equally common and pesty symptom. All these symptoms are at times referred to as morning sickness. Chances are, certain foods make you queasy even though you were used to eating them previously. The human body is extremely intuitive and if certain foods don't appeal to you or you crave foods that you never did before, it's a sign that your body wants something. If you are worried your baby is not getting sufficient nutrition, don't hesitate to consult your healthcare provider immediately. Here are some simple suggestions to manage nausea and food aversions.

The first thing you need to do is stay away from foods that have strong smells and spices such as garlic. Instead, look for alternatives to flavor the food you eat. If you have developed a newfound aversion to certain smells or strong smells that catch you off guard, the simplest way to counter this is by carrying a couple of fresh-cut slices of lemon with you. Simply sniff on them whenever a whiff of a strong smell bothers you. 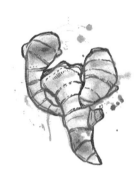 Try to incorporate some fresh ginger into your daily diet. Ginger not only regulates nausea but is good for your gut health as well. The natural antioxidants coupled with its refreshing flavor alleviates nausea. Sipping on fresh ginger tea, cooking with fresh ginger, eating ginger candies, or even sipping on ginger ale can be helpful.

As mentioned, avoid spices and foods with strong smells and instead opt for some bland foods such as toast, crackers, and even baked potatoes. If your prenatal vitamin is causing these symptoms, consult your healthcare provider and ask for something better. Remember, nutrition is important, and you might have to mask a couple of foods to ensure you are getting sufficient levels from them. For instance, simple vegetables such as carrots or other veggies can be sneaked into smoothies. Drinking a smoothie is simpler than eating a bowl full of food. Shift to liquids and smoothies for a while to reduce nausea.

Nausea and morning sickness can become a source of stress to an expecting mother, but this is just a temporary discomfort. These symptoms will not cause any developmental troubles for your baby. One thing that you cannot forget about is hydration. Dehydration is problematic.

Therefore, ensure that your body is thoroughly hydrated and that you are constantly sipping on different hydrating liquids such as broth, coconut water, ginger ale, or any other fluid that helps. If your body can tolerate it, don't discontinue a prenatal vitamin.

Heartburn

Pregnancy brings with it a variety of hormonal changes. As the pregnancy progresses, your baby is growing. Your body is also changing to accommodate the needs of this growing baby. As the baby pushes into the digestive organs to make more space for itself and the hormonal changes can trigger heartburn. This is an annoying side effect, but it can be easily managed. Ensure that you always sit upright after eating meals. Regardless of how tired you feel, don't give in to the temptation to lie down or rest for some time immediately after eating. Instead, sit for a while or try walking if possible. Avoid spicy, deep-fried, and extremely fatty foods and instead, replace them with bland and light meals. Other food items to avoid which bring about heartburn include caffeine, alcohol, spearmint, citrusy substances, and chocolate. Shift to eating smaller meals spaced throughout the day instead of three large ones. Also, make it a point to eat slowly. Apart from this, slowly sipping on a cold glass of milk mixed with some honey, snacking on almonds, and having a little ginger helps reduce heartburn.

Constipation

Any difficulty moving your bowels regularly is known as constipation. This is an extremely common symptom of pregnancy. This is due to the hormonal changes that take a toll on your digestive system along with the slowly expanding body catering to your growing baby's requirements. The hormones circulating in your body perform a variety of helpful functions during pregnancy, but it results in the relaxation of muscles, especially the ones in the digestive system. The good news is that you don't have to suffer from constipation or irregular and hard bowel movements. By focusing on some of the dietary suggestions given here, you can get ahead of constipation.

The first thing you need to do is consume foods rich in dietary fiber. The most common sources of it include fruits, vegetables, some types of beans, and whole grains. These natural sources offer the required fiber to make your bowel movements more regular. Adding some prunes to your daily diet is also a good idea because it's a natural laxative and helps reduce constipation. If your fiber intake increases, fluid intake should also increase. If you don't have sufficient fluids in the body or are dehydrated, your bowels become backed up. So, ensure that you are drinking plenty of water and other healthy fluids.

Another great way to tackle constipation is to add some form of physical activity to your daily routine. It doesn't mean you have to spend hours exercising vigorously. Instead, even walking a little every day does the trick. Anything that gets your body moving for as little as 20 minutes daily helps tackle constipation. If you have any worries or doubts about this, consult your healthcare provider about what you can do. Calcium supplements are commonly prescribed during pregnancy, and they are present in most multivitamins. It's also found in different foods, especially dairy products. Excess calcium intake results in constipation. It can also be caused by certain food sensitivities. So, if you notice that certain foods are making you constipated, stay away from them.

Start adding some probiotics to your daily diet. Probiotics refer to live helpful bacteria found in naturally fermented foods such as kimchi and yogurt. They support a healthy gut and in turn, promote better bowel movements and reduce constipation. Certain medicines also increase the risk of constipation. One such culprit is an iron supplement which is usually prescribed to prevent the risk of anemia. Some medications can also be used to tackle constipation, but they should be used only as a last resort. Please consult your healthcare provider for more information.

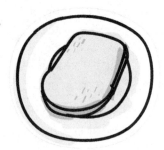

Your energy requirements will significantly increase during pregnancy. Growing a human within your body will obviously require more energy than usual. In normal cases, most usually have a cup of coffee or any other caffeinated beverage to feel fresh and energetic. Since this is no longer an option, focus on consuming energizing foods and making a few helpful lifestyle changes. An important change you must make is to ensure you are getting sufficient sleep. If you are unable to sleep properly at night, compensate for it with power naps during the day. However, regularizing your circadian rhythm and sleeping and waking up at consistent times is a better idea. You don't have to feel guilty or be hard on yourself if you notice you don't have the energy to do things you normally used to. Increase your intake of nutrient-dense and rich complex carbohydrates. Similarly, avoid sugar-rich foods because they cause spikes in energy levels that can leave you feeling tired. Another suggestion is to add some form of physical activity to your usual routine. Don't skip meals and whenever possible, opt for regularly spaced small meals.

Note: if any of these symptoms continue or you are worried about them, consult your healthcare provider immediately. Avoid using over-the-counter medicines and self-medication. Instead, only use those as prescribed by your doctor.

Pregnancy Diet Mistakes to Avoid

As important as it is to focus on nutrition, here are some common pregnancy diet mistakes you must avoid.

Supplements are only a means to bridge any nutritional gaps left behind in your usual diet. Don't think of them as a magic bullet to automatically obtain what your body needs. Instead, you need to focus on consuming wholesome and well-rounded meals. After all, you cannot meet your daily quota of needed macros by depending on supplements.

A healthy pregnancy diet is not synonymous with dieting instead, the focus should be on quality nutrition. Skipping meals can reduce your energy level and leave you feeling poorly. Don't skip meals to reduce your calorie intake or anything else along these lines. Right now, the primary focus should be to have a healthy pregnancy and ensure your growing baby obtains the required nutrients. If you are unable to eat large meals, opt for small meals that are regularly spaced throughout the day.

When it comes to a healthy pregnancy diet, it's not about how much you eat but what you eat that really matters. Stop prioritizing quantity over quality. You might have heard that you need to eat for two. It essentially means that the food you consume must cater to not just your body's energy requirements but to the growing baby as well.

Cravings are quite common during pregnancy and usually, cravings are an indicator that your body requires certain nutrients. If your usual diet before pregnancy was rich in unhealthy carbs, sugars, and salt or was a standard American diet, the chances are you start craving these things. Unfortunately, eating too many carbs, sugars, and other processed foods is extremely harmful. It increases inflammation, doesn't offer the required nutrients, and increases the risk of several problems such as eczema, gestational diabetes as well as acne.

To make things easier for yourself, you need to keep an open mind and start planning. A little planning and preparation go a long way when it comes to following a healthy diet. Following a healthy pregnancy, diet is not hard or expensive. By using the different recipes given in this book, you can rest easy knowing you are getting the daily dose of essential macro and micronutrients.

Key Takeaways

- A few healthy dietary and lifestyle changes will help manage any pregnancy symptoms you experience.

- Avoid spicy, fatty, and fried foods, and add bland foods to your diet to tackle morning sickness.

- Eat small meals and walk after eating to reduce heartburn.

- Increase the consumption of fiber-rich foods and fluids to regularize gut functioning and tackle constipation.

- Eat nutrient-dense and energizing foods and add some physical activity to your daily routine to overcome fatigue.

- Avoid skipping meals, consume nutrient-dense foods, plan your meals, and keep an open mind to ensure you are following a healthy pregnancy diet.

CHAPTER SEVEN

Breakfast, Lunch, Snack, Dinner, Side Dish, and Dessert Recipes

---

"Pregnancy can be a time when you take tremendous pleasure in eating, not only because you may enjoy food more but also because you know that it is nourishing both you and your baby."
Martha Rose and Jane L. Davis

Having the same menu, week after week during each trimester and after delivery would definitely be boring. Here are some recipes that you can choose from and make your own meal plan.

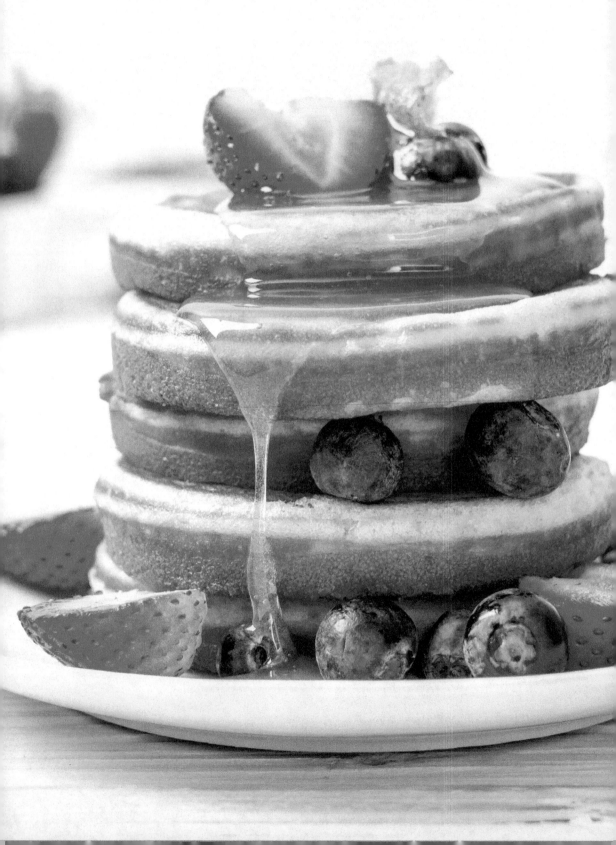

Breakfast

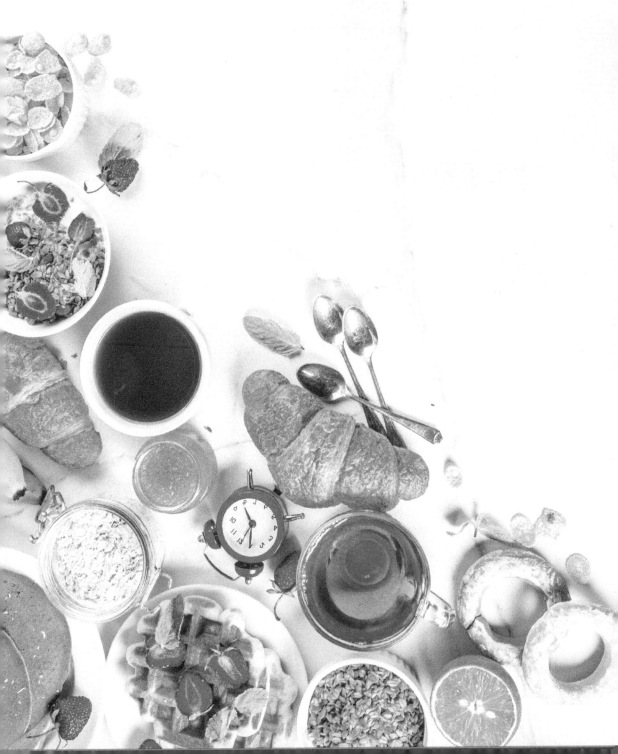

Chocolate Chip Banana Pancakes

Serves: 3

Nutritional values per serving: 1 pancake without serving options

Calories: 271

Fat: 16 g

Carbohydrate: 32 g

Protein: 5 g

Ingredients

- ½ large overripe banana, mashed
- 1 ½ tablespoons coconut oil, melted
- ¾ cup whole-wheat flour
- ¼ cup chocolate chips
- 1 tablespoon coconut sugar
- ½ cup coconut milk
- ½ teaspoon baking soda
- Serving options:
- Maple syrup, honey, agave syrup, or chocolate syrup
- Berries or fresh fruit of your choice
- Coconut butter or butter
- Jam or preserves
- Any other toppings of your choice

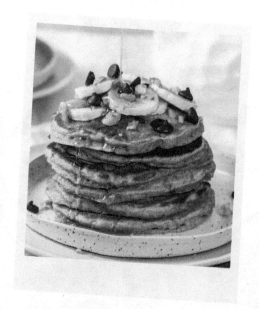

Directions

1. Add banana, sugar, milk, and oil into a bowl and mix until well incorporated.
2. Stir in the flour and baking soda. Stir until just incorporated. Do not over-mix
3. Add chocolate chips and fold gently.
4. Place a nonstick pan over medium heat. Spray the pan with cooking spray. When the pan is hot, scoop out 1/8 of the batter (about ¼ cup) and pour onto the pan.
5. Soon bubbles will start forming. Cook until the underside is brown in color. Turn the pancake over and cook the other side as well.
6. Remove the pancake from the pan and keep it warm.
7. Repeat steps 4-6 and make the remaining pancakes similarly.
8. Serve pancakes with suggested serving options.

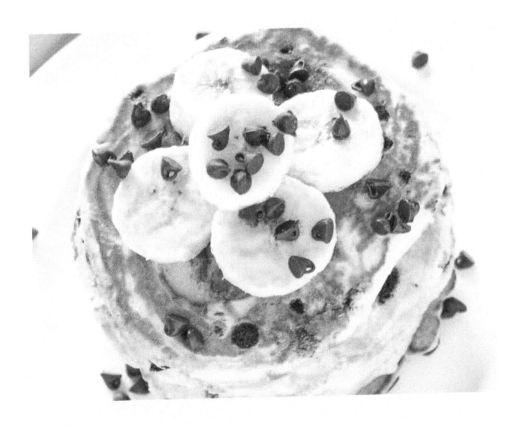

Fluffy Biscuits

Serves: 16

Nutritional values per serving: 1 biscuit

Calories: 249

Fat: 13 g

Carbohydrate: 26 g

Protein: 5 g

Ingredients

- 4 cups all-purpose flour
- 2 tablespoons sugar
- 1 cup shortening
- 1 1/8 cups 2% milk
- 8 teaspoons baking powder
- 1 teaspoon salt or to taste
- 2 large eggs, at room temperature

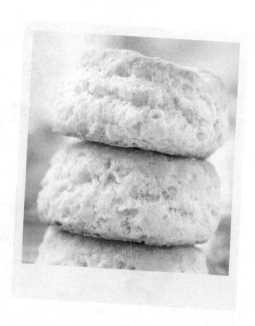

Directions

1. Set the temperature of the oven to 400° F and preheat the oven. Prepare 2–3 baking sheets by greasing lightly with cooking spray.
2. Combine flour, baking powder, sugar, and salt in a mixing bowl.
3. Add shortening and cut it into the mixture of dry ingredients until you get small crumbs.
4. Beat eggs and milk in a bowl and pour into the bowl of dry ingredients. Mix until just incorporated. You will get a moist dough.
5. Dust your countertop with a generous amount of flour. Place the dough on the floured area and knead about 10 times.
6. Dust your countertop if necessary. Roll the dough with a rolling pin until it is about ½ inch thick. Dust a biscuit cutter (2 ½ inches) with some flour and cut out biscuits from the dough.
7. Collect the scrap dough and repeat the previous step once again. You should get 16 biscuits in all.
8. Place the biscuits on the prepared baking sheets, leaving a sufficient gap between them.
9. Bake them in batches. Place a baking sheet in the oven and set the timer for 10 to 12 minutes or until golden brown.
10. Cool for a few minutes and serve.
11. Store leftover biscuits in freezer bags after cooling completely. Freeze until use. It can last for about 2 months.
12. To serve, reheat in a microwave and serve.

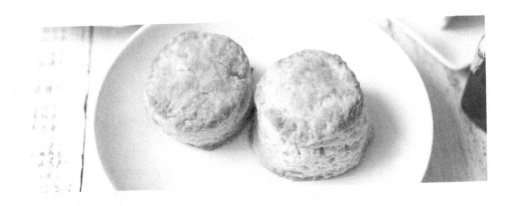

White Bean and Avocado Toast

Serves: 1

Nutritional values per serving:

Calories: 460

Fat: 18 g

Carbohydrate: 70 g

Protein: 22 g

Ingredients

- 2 slices whole-wheat bread
- 1 cup canned or cooked white beans, rinsed, drained
- Pepper to taste
- ½ cup mashed avocado
- Kosher salt to taste
- Crushed red pepper to taste

Directions

1. Mix together avocado and beans into a bowl.
2. Toast the bread slices to the desired doneness.
3. Spread avocado mixture over bread slices. Sprinkle salt, pepper, and crushed red pepper on top and serve.

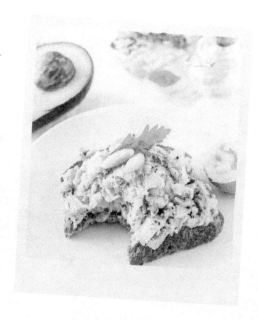

Chocolate Chip Banana Nut Muffins

Serves: 22

Nutritional values per serving: 1 muffin

Calories: 358

Fat: 17 g

Carbohydrate: 44 g

Protein: 11 g

Ingredients

- 2/3 cup canola oil
- 4 large eggs
- 6 medium ripe bananas
- 3 ½ cups whole-wheat flour
- 2 teaspoons baking soda
- 2 teaspoons ground cinnamon
- 1 cup chopped walnuts
- 4 scoops vanilla protein powder
- 1 teaspoon salt
- 2/3 cup rolled oats
- 1 cup honey
- 1 cup whole milk
- 2 teaspoons vanilla extract
- 1 ½ cups semi-sweet chocolate chips

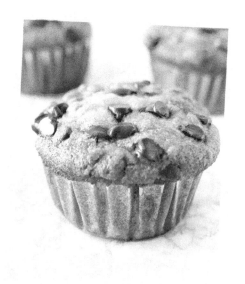

Directions

1. Set the temperature of the oven to 350° F and preheat the oven. Prepare 2 muffin pans of 12 cups each by greasing 22 of the cups with cooking spray. Place disposable liners if desired. I highly recommend disposable liners.
2. Add all the dry ingredients into a mixing bowl, i.e. flour, baking soda, oats, protein powder, and cinnamon.
3. Whisk together all the wet ingredients in another bowl, i.e. eggs, honey oil, and milk.
4. Add the wet ingredients into the bowl of dry ingredients and stir until well incorporated.
5. Add chocolate chips and walnuts and stir. Divide the batter into the prepared muffin cups.
6. Place the muffin pans in the oven and set the timer for 20 to 25 minutes or until cooked through. To check if the muffins are cooked, insert a toothpick in the center of the muffin and remove it. If you see any particles stuck on it, you need to bake for a few more minutes, else take out the muffin pans and let them cool.
7. Remove the muffins from the pan and serve. Store leftover muffins in an airtight container in the refrigerator. It can last for 8–10 days. You can also freeze them in freezer bags. They can last for two months.

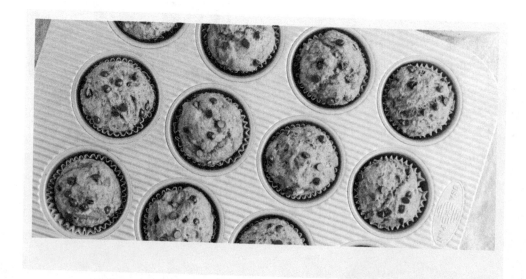

Breakfast Vegan Brownies

Serves: 12

Nutritional values per serving:

Calories: 145

Fat: 7.6 g

Carbohydrate: 15.3 g

Protein: 5.1 g

Ingredients

- ½ cup white whole-wheat flour
- 1 scoop plant-based protein powder
- ½ teaspoon salt
- 1 cup quick-cooking oats
- 2 tablespoons unsweetened cocoa powder
- ½ teaspoon baking soda
- 6 tablespoons brown sugar
- 1/8 cup canola oil
- ½ teaspoon vanilla extract
- 1 tablespoon flaxseed meal mixed with 3 tablespoons of water (this is 1 flax egg)
- 1/8 cup applesauce
- ½ tablespoon mini semi-sweet chocolate chips
- 1 tablespoon chopped nuts

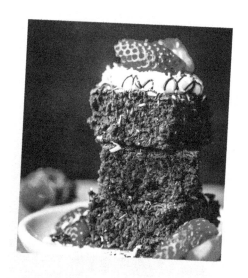

Directions

1. Once you mix up the flaxseed meal with water, place the bowl in the refrigerator for 15 minutes. It will be gel-like.
2. Set the temperature of the oven to 350° F and preheat the oven.
3. Prepare a small baking pan of about 6 inches by lining it with a sheet of parchment paper. Spray some cooking spray over the parchment paper.
4. Add all the dry ingredients into a bowl, i.e. flour, protein powder, salt, oats, cocoa, baking soda, and brown sugar, and stir.
5. Add all the wet ingredients into a mixing bowl, i.e. oil, vanilla, flax egg, and applesauce and whisk well.
6. Add the dry ingredients into the bowl of wet ingredients and mix until just combined.
7. Pour the batter into the prepared baking dish.
8. Sprinkle nuts and chocolate chips on top.
9. Place the baking dish in the oven and set the timer for about 15-20 minutes or until cooked through. To check if the brownies are cooked, insert a toothpick in the center of the brownie and remove it. If you see any particles stuck on it, you need to bake for a few more minutes, otherwise take out the baking dish and let it cool.
10. Cut into 12 equal squares. Store leftover brownies in an airtight container in the refrigerator. It can last for 8–10 days. You can also freeze them in freezer bags. They can last for 2 months.

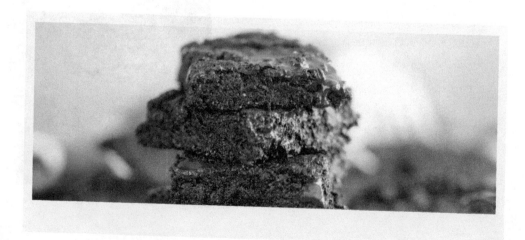

Cranberry Nut Granola Bars

Serves: 12

Nutritional values per serving:

Calories: 169

Fat: 7.5 g

Carbohydrate: 22.3 g

Protein: 4.8 g

Ingredients

- ½ cup old-fashioned oats
- 1 cup quick-cooking oats
- ¼ cup hulled pumpkin seeds
- ½ cup mixed nuts
- ½ can (from a 14 ounces can) sweetened condensed milk
- ¼ cup slivered almonds
- ½ cup dried cranberries

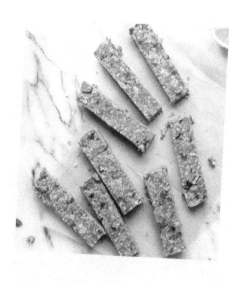

Directions

1. Set the temperature of the oven to 350° F and preheat the oven. Prepare a small, square baking dish (about 6 inches) by lining it with a large sheet of parchment paper such that slightly overhangs. This helps for the easy removal of the bars after baking.
2. Lightly spray the parchment paper with some oil.
3. Add pumpkin seeds, almonds, mixed nuts, condensed milk, cranberries, and all the oats into a mixing bowl and mix well.
4. Spoon the mixture into the baking dish. Spread it evenly and press it onto the bottom of the baking dish.
5. Put the baking dish into the oven and set the timer for 20 to 25 minutes or until it is golden brown around the edges. If you like chewy bars, bake for 20 minutes, and if you like crunchy bars, bake for 25 minutes.
6. Let the bars cool for 5 minutes.
7. Lift the bars out with the help of the overhanging parchment paper.
8. Take a sharp knife and cut into 12 equal bars.
9. Store leftover bars in an airtight container at room temperature or in the refrigerator. It can last for 8–10 days in the refrigerator and about 3–4 days at room temperature.

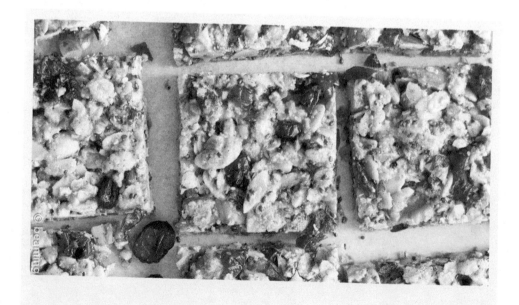

Snack

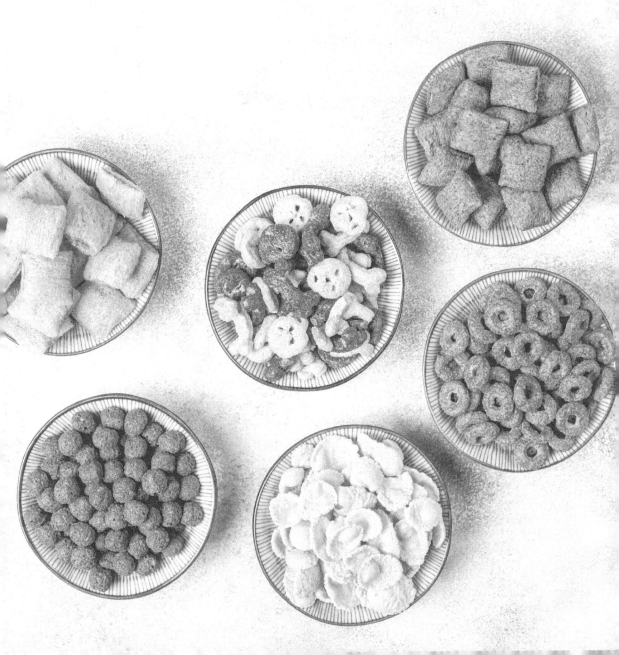

No-Bake Peanut Butter Cookies

Serves: 24

Nutritional values per serving:

Calories: 192

Fat: 11.16 g

Carbohydrate: 25.48 g

Protein: 6.61 g

Ingredients

- 1 1/8 cups unsalted natural creamy peanut butter
- 4 tablespoons melted coconut oil
- 1 ¼ teaspoons sea salt
- ½ cup mini chocolate chips
- 1 cup maple syrup
- 2 teaspoons vanilla extract
- 5 cups rolled oats

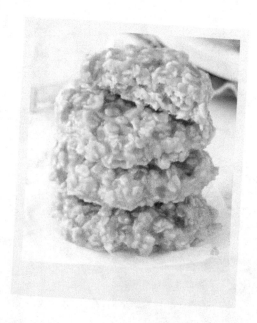

Directions

1. Prepare a large baking sheet by lining it with parchment paper.
2. Add maple syrup, peanut butter, coconut oil, salt, and vanilla into a bowl and whisk until very smooth.
3. Stir in the oats and chocolate chips. Mix until well incorporated.
4. Make 24 equal portions of the mixture and shape them into balls. You should get about 2 tablespoons of mixture per ball.
5. Place them on the prepared baking sheet, leaving a sufficient gap between them. Now press the balls until slightly flat, to the desired thickness.
6. Place the baking sheet in the refrigerator and let it chill for at least 8–9 hours or until firm.
7. Transfer the cookies into an airtight container and chill until use. It can last for 3–4 weeks.

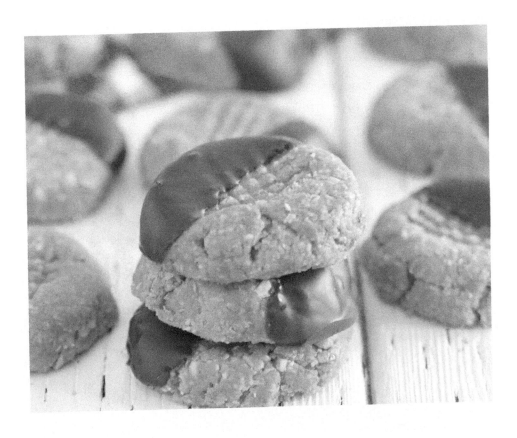

Breaded Chicken Fingers

Serves: 4

Nutritional values per serving:

Calories: 345

Fat: 15.7 g

Carbohydrate: 24.6 g

Protein: 25.4 g

Ingredients

- 3 boneless, skinless chicken breast halves, cut into ½ inch steps
- ½ cup buttermilk
- ½ cup all-purpose flour
- ½ teaspoon salt
- Oil to fry, as required
- 2 small eggs, beaten
- ¾ teaspoon garlic powder
- ½ cup seasoned breadcrumbs
- ½ teaspoon baking powder

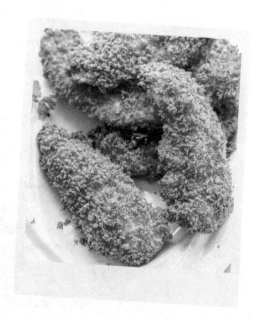

Directions

1. Beat eggs, garlic, and buttermilk in a bowl. Add chicken into a Ziploc bag. Pour the egg mixture into the bag and seal the bag. Turn the bag around a few times so that chicken is well coated with the mixture.
2. Place the bag in the refrigerator for 2–4 hours.
3. Combine flour, baking powder, salt, and breadcrumbs in a bowl.
4. Take out the chicken from the bag and discard the marinade.
5. Dredge chicken in the flour mixture.
6. Pour oil into a deep frying pan, such that it is about 2 inches in height from the bottom of the pan.
7. Heat the oil until it is very hot but not smoking, around 365° F.
8. Fry the chicken in batches until golden brown.
9. Remove chicken with a slotted spoon and place on a plate lined with paper towels.
10. Serve with a dip of your choice.

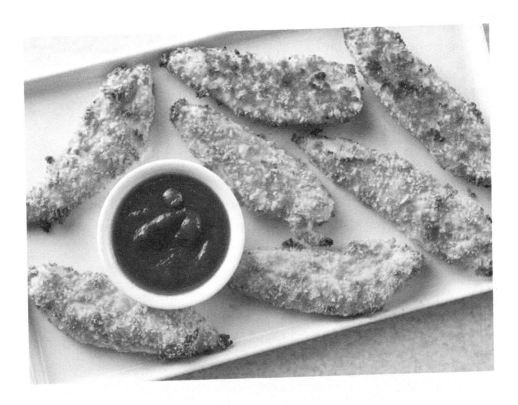

Avocado Fries

Serves: 3

Nutritional values per serving:

Calories: 330

Fat: 24 g

Carbohydrate: 25 g

Protein: 5 g

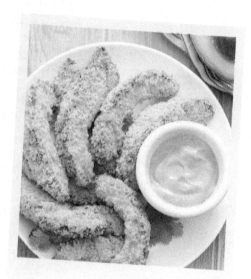

Ingredients

- 1 large firm avocado, peeled, cut into ½ inch thick slices
- ½ tablespoon chili powder
- 1 egg, beaten
- 3 tablespoons vegetable oil
- ¾ cup panko breadcrumbs
- ¼ cup all-purpose flour
- 1 teaspoon salt, divided

Directions

1. Add flour, ½ teaspoon salt, and chili powder into a bowl and mix well.
2. Coat the avocado slices in the flour mixture, one at a time, then dip it in egg, and finally dredge in panko breadcrumbs.
3. Pour oil into a large pan and let it heat over medium-high heat. When the oil is hot, add the avocado slices to the pan. Spread them in a single layer, without overlapping.
4. Cook until the underside is golden brown. Turn the slices over and cook the other side for a few minutes until the underside is golden brown.
5. Remove avocado slices with a slotted spoon and place them on a plate lined with paper towels.
6. Serve with a dip of your choice.

Clam Fritter Snacks

Serves: 8

Nutritional values per serving:

Calories: 304

Fat: 21.6 g

Carbohydrate: 22.2 g

Protein: 21.6 g

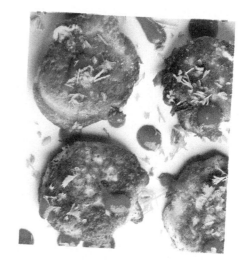

Ingredients

- 2 cans (10 ounces each) minced clams, drained
- 2 eggs, beaten
- 2 cups baking mix
- 4 tablespoons vegetable oil

Directions

1. Beat eggs in a bowl. Add baking mix and mix well.
2. Add clams and mix well.
3. Pour half the oil into a large pan and let it heat over medium-high heat. When the oil is hot, add half the clam into the pan. Spread them in a single layer, without overlapping.
4. Cook until the underside is golden brown. Turn the clams over and cook the other side for a few minutes until the underside is golden brown.
5. Remove clams with a slotted spoon and place them on a plate lined with paper towels.
6. Serve with a dip of your choice.

Peanut Butter Popcorn

Serves: 4

Nutritional values per serving:

Calories: 181

Fat: 22.3 g

Carbohydrate: 43.9 g

Protein: 4.7 g

Ingredients

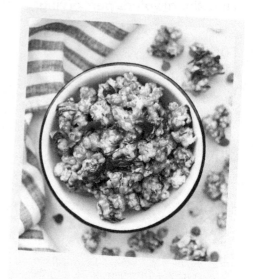

- 1 package (3.5 ounces) microwave popcorn
- 6 tablespoons brown sugar
- 10 large marshmallows
- ¼ cup margarine
- 2 tablespoons peanut butter

Directions

1. Pop the popcorn following the directions given on the package.
2. Place popcorn in a large bowl.
3. Add brown sugar, margarine, and marshmallows into a microwave-safe bowl. Cook on high for about 2 minutes or until the mixture melts and is smooth. Stir the mixture every 40–45 seconds while melting.
4. Add peanut butter and mix well. Drizzle the melted peanut butter mixture over the popcorn and stir immediately.
5. You can serve it right away or cool it for a few minutes and serve.

Feta 'n' Chive Muffins

Serves: 6

Nutritional values per serving:

Calories: 105

Fat: 4 g

Carbohydrate: 13 g

Protein: 4 g

Ingredients

- ¾ cup all-purpose flour
- 1/8 teaspoon salt or to taste
- ½ cup fat-free milk
- ¼ cup crumbled feta cheese
- 1 ½ teaspoons baking powder
- 1 large egg, at room temperature
- 1 tablespoon butter, melted
- 1 ½ tablespoons minced chives

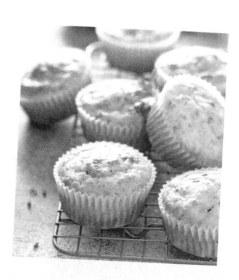

Directions

1. Set the temperature of the oven to 350° F and preheat the oven. Prepare a 6 cup muffin pan by greasing it with cooking spray. Line the cups with paper liners if desired.
2. Add flour, salt, and baking powder into a bowl and stir until well combined.
3. Whisk together milk, egg, and butter in another bowl.
4. Pour the milk mixture into the bowl of the flour mixture and stir until just incorporated, making sure not to over-mix.
5. Add feta cheese and chives and fold gently.
6. Spoon the batter into the muffin cups. Place the muffin pan in the oven and set the timer for 20–25 minutes or until the muffins are cooked through.
7. To check if the muffins are cooked, insert a toothpick in the center of the muffin and remove it. If you see any particles stuck on it, you need to bake for a few more minutes, otherwise take out the muffin pans and let them cool.
8. Remove the muffins from the pan and serve. Store leftover muffins in an airtight container in the refrigerator. It can last for 4–5 days. You can also freeze them in freezer bags. They can last for 2 months.

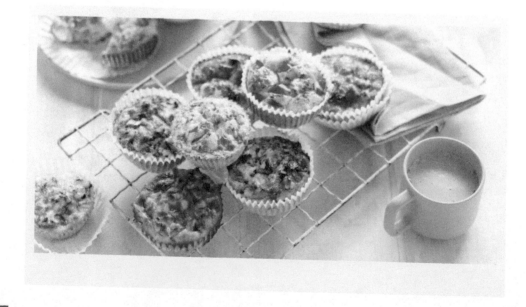

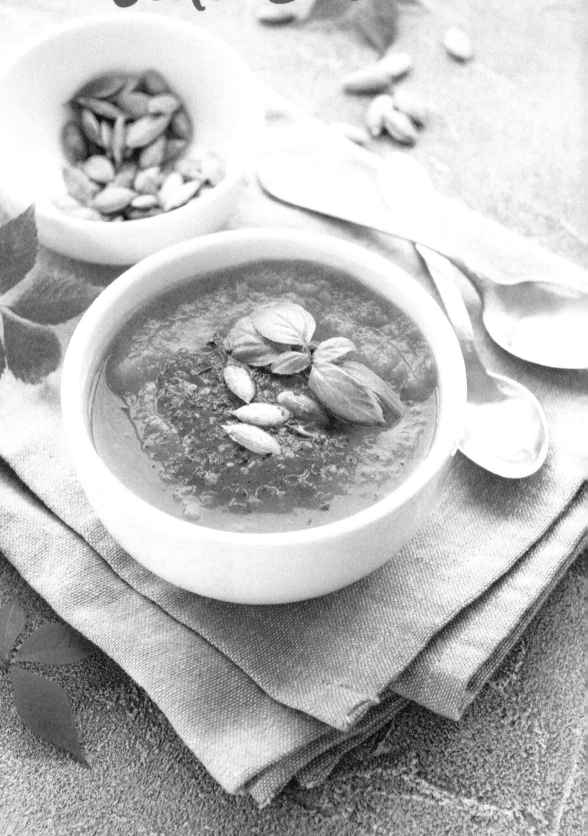

Onion Rings

Serves: 3

Nutritional values per serving:

Calories: 289

Fat: 15 g

Carbohydrate: 33 g

Protein: 4 g

Ingredients

- ½ pound large onions
- Oil to fry, as required
- 3 tablespoons cornstarch
- For the batter:
- ¾ cup + 1 tablespoon flour
- 1 teaspoon paprika
- 1 teaspoon salt
- 6 ounces beer
- ½ teaspoon baking powder
- ½ teaspoon garlic powder
- ¼ teaspoon pepper or to taste

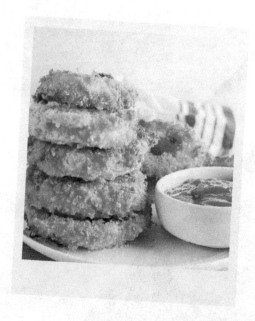

1. Place onions in a bowl of ice water for 15 minutes. Dry them with a clean towel.
2. Now peel and cut the onions into round slices. Separate the rings.
3. Place the rings on a plate and sprinkle cornstarch over the rings.
4. To make, combine ¾ cup flour, paprika, baking powder, pepper, garlic powder, and salt in a bowl.
5. Add beer and stir constantly until smooth. You should have a pancake-like batter. If necessary, add the remaining 1 tablespoon of flour or more if required.
6. Pour oil into a deep frying pan, such that it is about 2 inches in height from the bottom of the pan.
7. Heat the oil until it is very hot but not smoking, around 375° F.
8. Dip 4 to 5 rings in the batter and slide them carefully into the hot oil, one at a time. Cook until golden brown.
9. Remove the onion rings with a slotted spoon and place them on a plate lined with paper towels. Fry the remaining onion rings in batches.

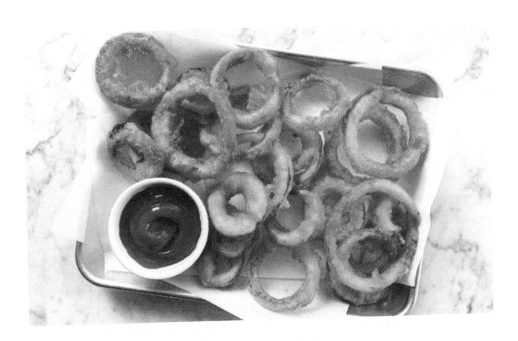

Coleslaw

Serves: 3
Nutritional values per serving:
Calories: 160
Fat: 14 g
Carbohydrate: 8 g
Protein: 1 g

Ingredients

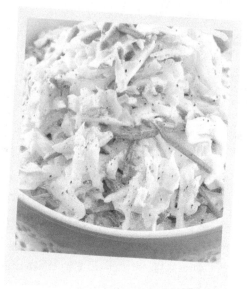

- 1 cup finely shredded purple cabbage
- 1 ½ cups finely shredded green cabbage
- ½ cup finely shredded carrot
- For dressing:
- ½ tablespoon white vinegar
- 1 teaspoon sugar
- 1 teaspoon cider vinegar
- Salt to taste
- ¼ cup mayonnaise
- ¼ teaspoon celery seeds
- Pepper to taste

Directions

1. To make the dressing: Add white vinegar, sugar, cider vinegar, salt, mayonnaise, celery seeds, and pepper into a bowl and whisk well.
2. Add cabbage and carrot and mix well.

Parsnip, Pear and Pecan Salad

Serves: 4

Nutritional values per serving:

Calories: 254

Fat: 20 g

Carbohydrate: 14 g

Protein: 7 g

Ingredients

- ½ cup shredded parmesan cheese
- ½ cup cubed pears
- ¼ cup fresh or frozen peas, thawed if frozen
- ¼ cup pine nuts
- ¼ teaspoon pepper
- 1 ½ - 2 tablespoons water
- 1 cup julienne-cut parsnip
- ¼ cup chopped pecans
- ¼ cup pomegranate seeds
- ½ teaspoon kosher salt
- 3 tablespoons mayonnaise

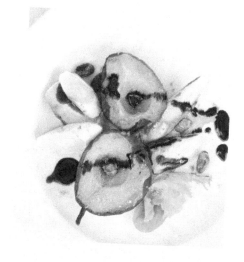

Directions

1. Set the temperature of the oven to 400° F and preheat the oven.
2. Prepare a baking sheet by lining it with parchment paper. Take 2 tablespoons of the parmesan cheese and drop it on the baking sheet, in a heap. So you should have 4 heaps of cheese. Leave sufficient gaps between them.
3. Place the baking sheet in the oven and set the timer for 12 minutes or until the cheese melts and the rounds turn golden brown. Let it cool to room temperature.
4. Add pears, peas, pine nuts, pepper, water, parsnip, pecans, pomegranate, salt, and mayonnaise into a bowl and mix well.
5. Divide salt into 4 plates. Serve each plate with a parmesan crisp.

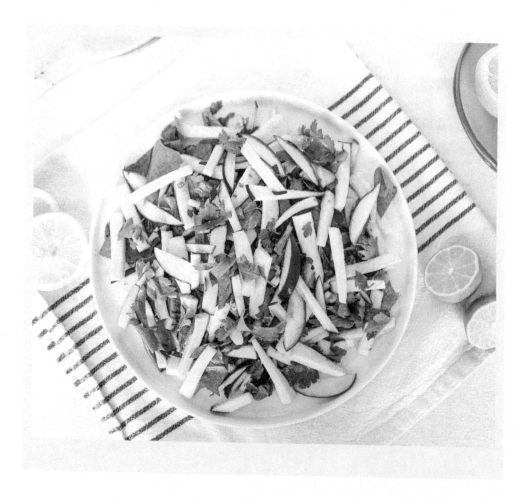

Apple, Walnut and Potato Gratin

Serves: 5

Nutritional values per serving:

Calories: 171

Fat: 8.4 g

Carbohydrate: 19.6 g

Protein: 6 g

Ingredients

- ½ cup milk
- 1.1 pounds desiree potatoes, peeled, cut into thin slices
- 2 tablespoons crumbled gorgonzola cheese
- ¼ cup chopped walnuts
- 1 clove garlic, crushed
- 1 large golden delicious apple, cored, peeled, cut into thin slices
- ¼ cup grated cheddar cheese

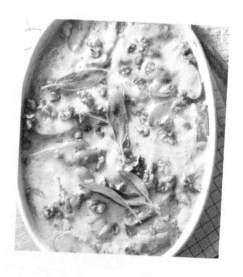

Directions

1. Set the temperature of the oven to 400° F and preheat the oven. Prepare a small baking dish by greasing it with cooking spray.
2. Bring garlic and milk to a simmer in a saucepan over medium-low heat. Turn off the heat.
3. Place alternate slices of potato and apple in the baking dish. Insert cheese crumbs in between the slices.
4. Remove the garlic and pour over the apple and potato slices. Keep the baking dish covered with foil.
5. Put the baking dish in the oven and set the timer for about 45–60 minutes.
6. Once the potato slices are cooked, cool for 5 minutes and serve.

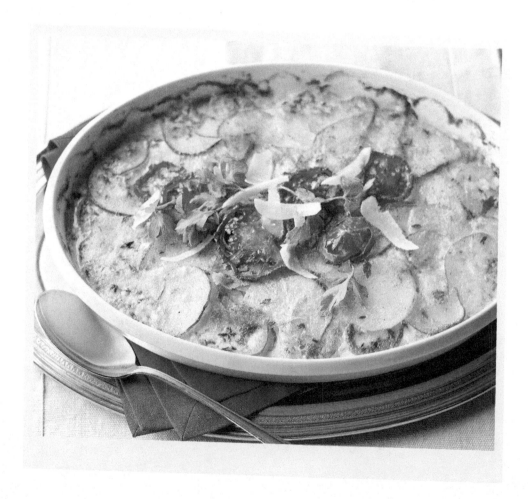

Ginger and Apricot Salad

Serves: 2

Nutritional values per serving:

Calories: 181

Fat: 3 g

Carbohydrate: 40 g

Protein: 5 g

Ingredients

- ½ can (from a 16 ounces can) apricot halves, drained
- ½ teaspoon sugar
- 2 small cloves garlic, minced
- 1/8 teaspoon pepper or to taste
- 2 ½ cups mixed salad greens
- ¾ pound fresh green beans, trimmed, cut into 3 inch pieces
- 2 tablespoons rice vinegar
- ¼ teaspoon minced fresh ginger
- 1/8 teaspoon salt
- 1 ½ tablespoons coarsely chopped roasted peanuts
- ½ medium mango, peeled, chopped

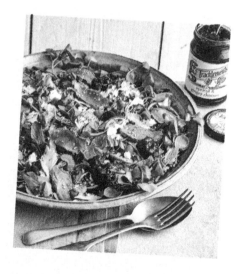

Directions

1. Add apricot, vinegar, sugar, ginger, garlic, salt, and pepper into a blender and blend until smooth.
2. Boil a pot of water over high heat. Drop the beans into the boiling water and cook until the beans are tender and have a crunch.
3. Drain the beans and immerse them in ice water. Dry the beans with a towel and add to a bowl.
4. Add mango and salad greens and toss well. Drizzle the dressing over the salad. Toss well and serve.

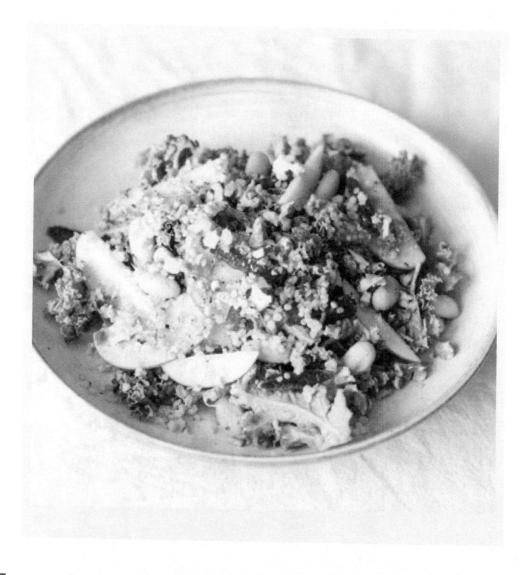

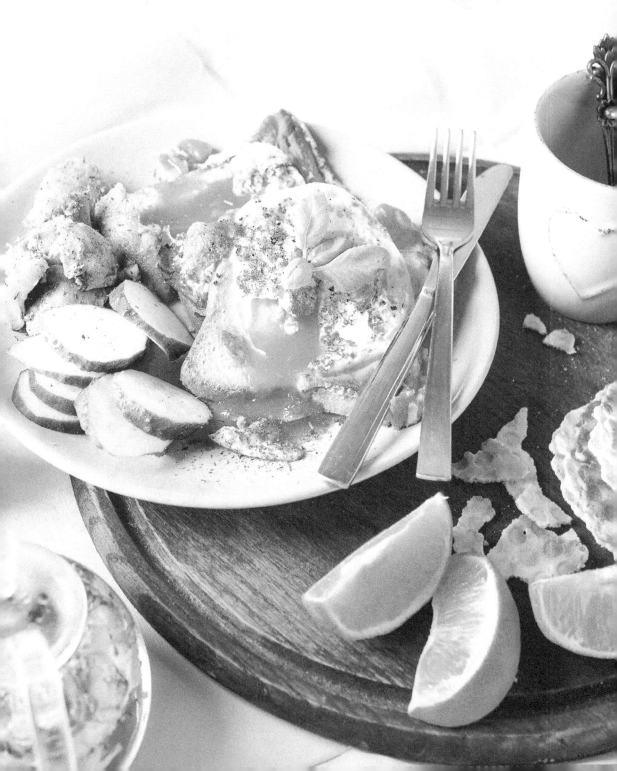

Lunch

Spinach and Dill Pasta Salad

Serves: 2

Nutritional values per serving:

Calories: 367

Fat: 19 g

Carbohydrate: 41 g

Protein: 12 g

Ingredients

For dressing:

- 2 tablespoons white wine vinegar
- ½ teaspoon dried dill
- Salt to taste
- 2 tablespoons extra-virgin olive oil
- Pepper to taste

For salad:

- 1 ½ cups cooked whole-wheat fusilli or penne pasta
- 1 cup halved cherry tomatoes
- ¼ cup shredded cheese
- 2 cups chopped spinach
- ½ cup edamame, thawed if frozen
- 1 small red onion, finely chopped

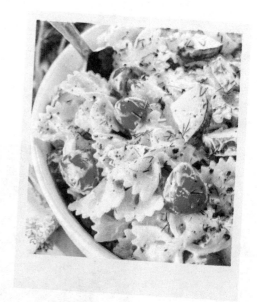

Directions

1. To make the dressing: Add vinegar, dill, salt, oil, and pepper into a bowl and whisk well. Set aside for a while for the flavors to set in.
2. To make the salad: Add pasta, tomatoes, cheese, spinach, edamame, and onion into a bowl. Toss well.
3. Pour dressing on top. Toss well and serve.

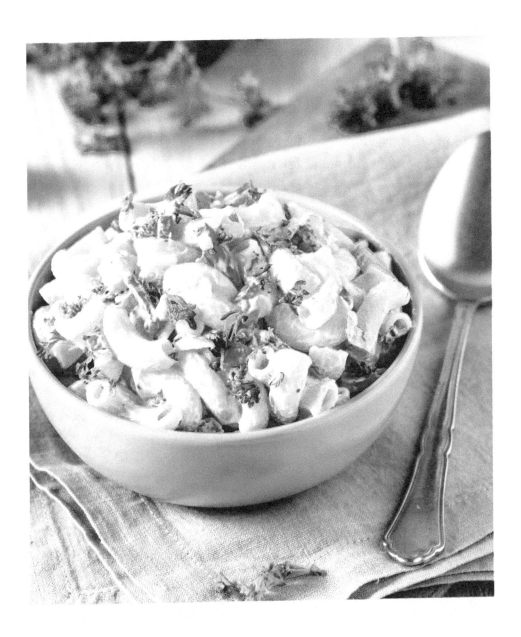

Roasted Asparagus Risotto

Serves: 4

Nutritional values per serving:

Calories: 311

Fat: 7 g

Carbohydrate: 44 g

Protein: 16 g

Ingredients

- 1 pound fresh asparagus, cut into 1 inch pieces
- 2 ½ - 3 cups low-sodium chicken broth
- 1 clove garlic, minced
- 1 cup uncooked Arborio rice
- ¼ teaspoon pepper or to taste
- 6 thin slice prosciutto
- ½ shallot, chopped
- 1 teaspoon olive oil
- ¼ cup white wine
- ½ cup grated parmesan cheese

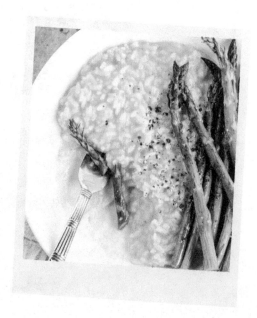

Directions

1. Set the temperature of the oven to 400° F and preheat the oven.
2. Put the asparagus on a baking sheet and put it in the oven. Set the timer for about 25 minutes or until they are tender with a crisp in it.
3. Take a baking dish and place the prosciutto in it. Put it into the oven and set the timer for about 10 minutes or until crisp.
4. When it cools, crumble the prosciutto.
5. Warm the broth in a saucepan and let it remain on low heat on your stovetop.
6. Pour oil into a skillet and place it over medium heat. When the oil is hot, add shallot and garlic and cook until slightly soft.
7. Stir in rice and cook for a couple of minutes. Turn down the heat to low heat.
8. Add pepper and wine and stir. Cook until dry. Pour ½ cup of the simmering broth and cook until dry. Repeat this adding of broth and each time cook until dry. Cook until the rice is tender.
9. Stir in prosciutto, asparagus, and cheese. Heat thoroughly and serve.

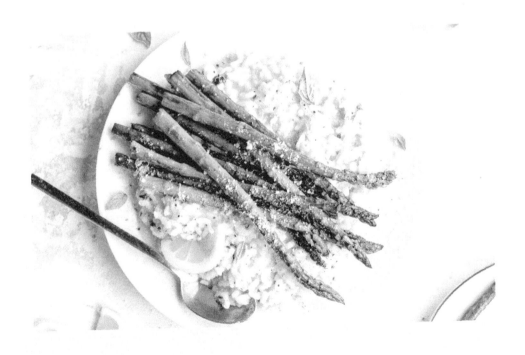

Edamame Hummus Wrap

Serves: 2

Nutritional values per serving:

Calories: 339

Fat: 20 g

Carbohydrate: 35 g

Protein: 14 g

Ingredients

- 6 ounces frozen shelled edamame, thawed
- 1 ½ tablespoons extra-virgin olive oil, divided
- 2 small cloves garlic, chopped
- Pepper to taste
- 1 cup very thinly sliced green cabbage
- ½ scallion, thinly sliced
- 2 spinach or whole-wheat tortillas (8 inches each)
- 3 tablespoons lemon juice, divided
- 1 tablespoon tahini
- ¼ teaspoon ground cumin
- ¼ teaspoon salt or to taste
- ¼ cup sliced orange bell pepper
- A handful fresh parsley, chopped

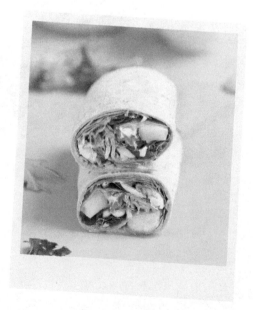

1. To make edamame hummus:: Add edamame, 1 tablespoon oil, 1 ½ tablespoons lemon juice, salt, pepper, cumin, garlic, and tahini into the food processor bowl and process until smooth.
2. Pour the hummus into a bowl.
3. Add pepper, ½ tablespoon of oil, and lemon juice into another bowl and whisk well. Stir in the bell pepper, cabbage, parsley, and scallion. Mix until well coated.
4. Place tortillas on your countertop. Smear about ½ of the edamame hummus over it on 1/8 of the lower portion of the tortilla.
5. Spread ½ of the cabbage mixture over the hummus.
6. Roll like a burrito and serve.

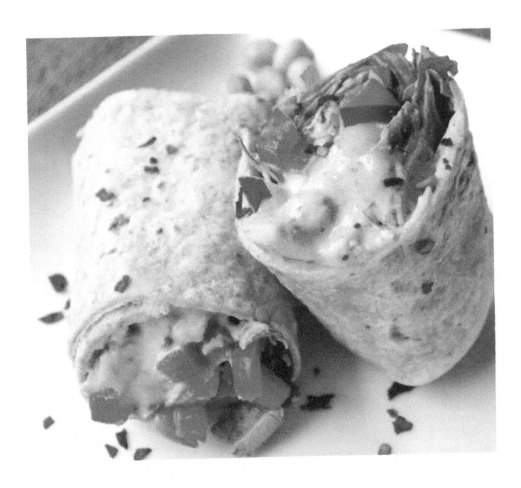

Healthy Lentil Soup

Serves: 2

Nutritional values per serving:

Calories: 323

Fat: 8 g

Carbohydrate: 47 g

Protein: 21 g

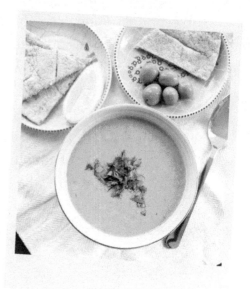

Ingredients

- ½ teaspoon vegetable oil
- ½ carrot, sliced
- ½ onion, chopped
- ½ cup brown dry lentils, rinsed, soaked in water for 1–2 hours
- 1 bay leaf
- ½ tablespoons lemon juice (optional)
- 2 cups vegetable broth
- 1/8 teaspoon dried thyme
- Salt to taste
- Pepper to taste

Directions

1. Pour oil into a soup pot and let it heat over medium heat. When the oil is hot, add onion and carrot and cook until onions turns translucent.
2. Add lentils, bay leaf, broth, thyme, salt, and pepper and stir.
3. When it begins to boil, lower the heat and cover with a lid. Simmer until the lentils are soft. Discard the bay leaf.
4. Add lemon juice just before serving and stir.
5. Ladle the soup into soup bowls and serve.
6. You could cook the lentils in a pressure cooker or instant pot as it is much quicker.

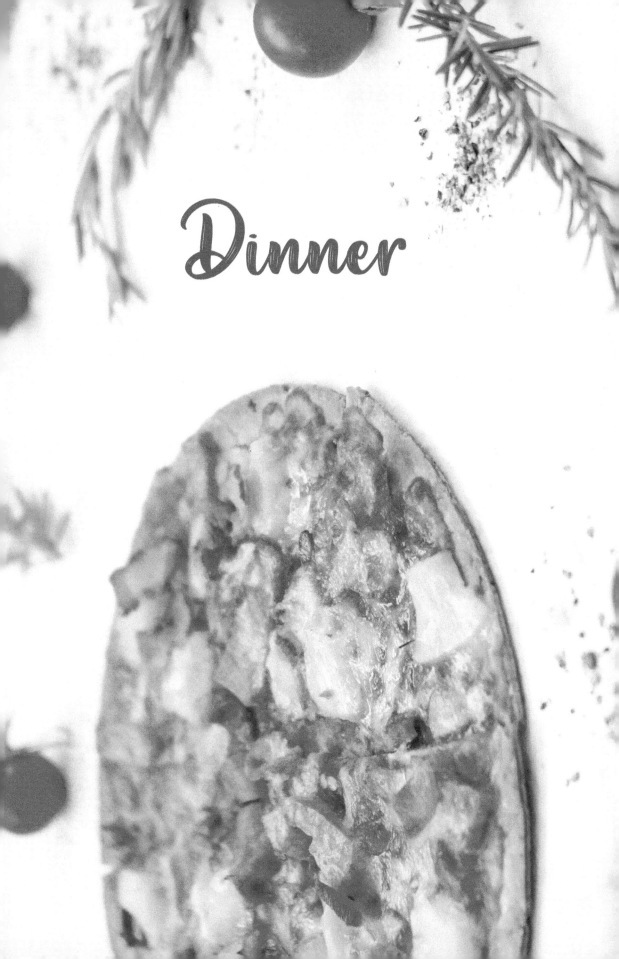

Dinner

Arugula and Brown Rice Salad

Serves: 2

Nutritional values per serving:

Calories: 473

Fat: 22 g

Carbohydrate: 53 g

Protein: 13 g

For the salad:

- ½ package (from an 8.8 ounces package) ready-to serve brown rice
- ½ can (from a 15 ounces can chickpeas, rinsed, drained
- 1/8 cup loosely packed fresh basil leaves, torn
- 2 ½ cups fresh arugula or baby spinach
- ½ cup crumbled feta cheese
- ¼ cup dried cherries or cranberries

For the dressing:

- 2 tablespoons olive oil
- 1 tablespoon lemon juice
- Pepper to taste
- 1/8 teaspoon grated lemon zest
- Salt to taste

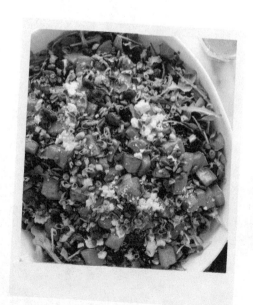

Directions

1. Warm up the rice following the directions given on the package.
2. Let the rice cool for a few minutes, until warm.
3. Add rice, beans, arugula, cherries, cheese, and basil into a bowl and mix well.
4. To make the dressing: Add oil, lemon juice, pepper, lemon zest, and salt into a bowl and whisk well. Pour the dressing over the salad. Toss well and serve.

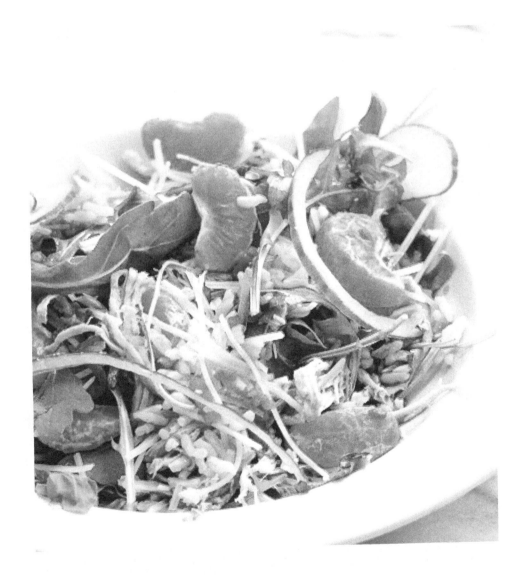

Mushroom Risotto

Serves: 2

Nutritional values per serving:

Calories: 349

Fat: 8.7 g

Carbohydrate: 50.2 g

Protein: 12.8 g

Ingredients

- ½ ounce dried porcini mushrooms
- 2 teaspoons extra-virgin olive oil, divided
- ½ cup short grain brown rice
- ½ tablespoon chopped fresh thyme or ½ teaspoon dried thyme
- 1 ½ cups chicken broth
- ¼ cup freshly grated parmesan cheese
- 1 teaspoon balsamic vinegar
- Freshly ground pepper to taste
- ¾ cup hot water
- ½ cup sliced leek
- 1 clove garlic, minced
- ¼ cup dry white wine
- 2 ounces cremini mushrooms or baby Bella mushrooms
- 1/8 cup freshly chopped parsley or to taste
- Salt to taste

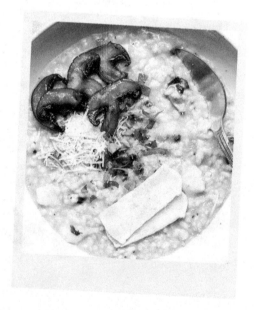

1. Soak porcini mushrooms in hot water. Let it rehydrate for 30 minutes.
2. Strain the mushrooms but retain the soaking liquid.
3. Rinse the mushrooms well and drain them in a colander.
4. Chop the rehydrated mushrooms into fine pieces.
5. Set the temperature of the oven to 425° F and preheat the oven.
6. Pour 1 teaspoon of oil into an ovenproof skillet and place it over medium heat. When the oil is hot, add porcini and leek and cook until tender. Stir frequently.
7. Cook for a couple of minutes. Stir in thyme, garlic, and rice. Stir for a minute or so until the rice is well combined with the leek mixture.
8. Stir in the broth and cook until nearly dry. Then stir in the soaked mushroom liquid.
9. When it starts boiling, turn off the heat. Keep the pan covered and shift the pan into the oven.
10. Set the timer for about 40 minutes or until the rice is tender. If there is too much liquid in the pan and the rice is cooked, shift the pan onto the stovetop and cook until dry or the way you prefer it to be cooked.
11. Meanwhile, pour the remaining oil into a skillet and let it heat over medium-high heat.
12. When the oil is hot, add cremini mushrooms and mix well. Cook until brown.
13. Add cremini mushrooms, half the parsley, parmesan cheese, salt, vinegar, and pepper mix well.
14. Garnish with remaining parsley and serve.

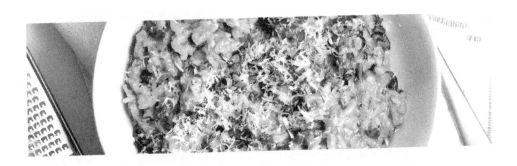

Lamb Chops with Pear and Balsamic Pan Sauce

Serves: 4

Serves:

Nutritional values per serving: 2 lamb chops with ¼ pear and 2 tablespoons sauce

Calories: 230

Fat: 6 g

Carbohydrate: 11 g

Protein: 31 g

Ingredients

- 8 medium lamb loin chops (¾ inch thick), trimmed of fat
- ½ teaspoon pepper
- ½ cup low-sodium beef broth
- 1 ripe, firm pear, peeled, cored, and cut into ¼ inch thick slices
- ½ teaspoon fine sea salt
- ½ cup unsweetened pure apple juice
- 3 teaspoons balsamic vinegar
- 1 ½ teaspoons chopped fresh rosemary or thyme or a mixture of both + extra to serve

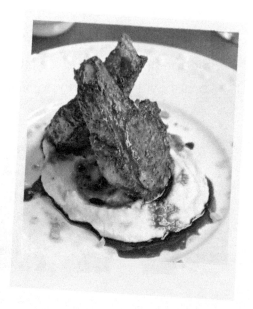

Directions

1. Place a nonstick skillet over medium-high heat. Season the lamb chops with salt and pepper and place them in the skillet.
2. Cook for 2 ½ minutes on each side for medium-rare or 4 minutes on each side for medium cooked. Remove lamb with a slotted spoon and place on a plate.
3. Cover and set aside.
4. Drain off the fat that is remaining in the skillet. Turn down the heat to medium heat.
5. Add pears, apple juice, broth, and vinegar. Scrape the bottom of the skillet to remove any browned bits that are stuck.
6. Simmer until the liquid in the pan is boiled down to half its original quantity. Turn off the heat and add the rosemary.
7. Place lamb on individual serving plates. Divide the pear slices equally and place them over the lamb. Pour sauce on top.
8. Garnish with some fresh herbs if desired and serve.

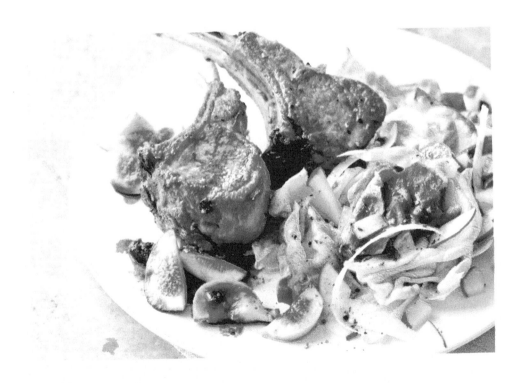

Potato Curry

Serves: 3

Nutritional values per serving:

Calories: 452

Fat: 17.5 g

Carbohydrate: 65.5 g

Protein: 10.6 g

Ingredients

- 6 new potatoes
- ½ cup frozen green peas
- 1 tablespoon tomato paste
- 3 tablespoons cashews, soaked in water for 15 minutes, drained, chopped
- 1 cup cherry tomatoes
- ¼ teaspoon ground cumin
- A handful fresh cilantro, chopped
- ½ tablespoon olive oil
- Salt to taste
- 1/8 teaspoon cayenne pepper or to taste
- Pepper to taste
- ½ can (from a 14 ounces can) coconut milk
- 5-6 basil leaves, chopped
- ¼ cup water

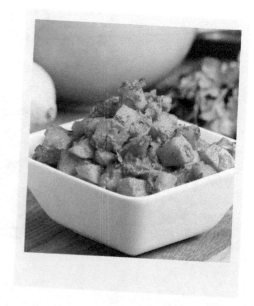

Directions

1. Cook potatoes in a small pot filled with water over medium-high heat until soft. Drain and set aside.
2. Place a pan over medium heat. Roast the cashews for 4-5 minutes.
3. Add potatoes and stir. Stir in the tomatoes, spices, tomato paste, and water.
4. Lower the heat and simmer until the tomatoes are slightly soft.
5. Stir in the peas and coconut milk and cook until the gravy is thick. Add salt and pepper to taste. Turn off the heat.
6. Garnish with basil and serve over rice or quinoa or any other grains of your choice.

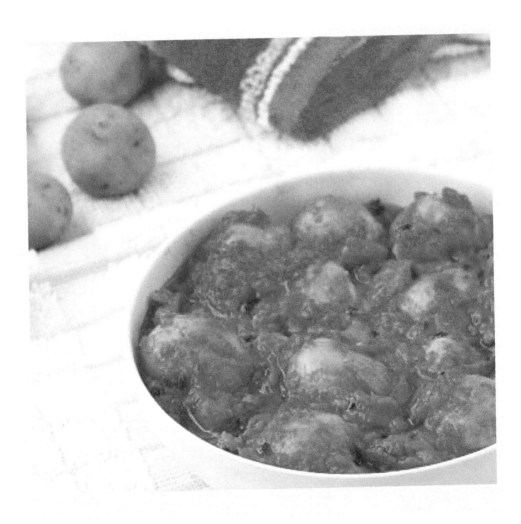

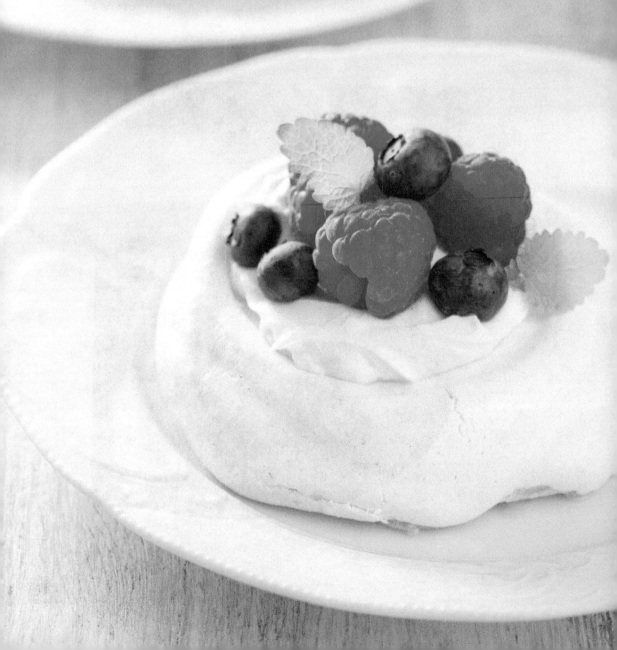

Dessert

Fruit Salsa and Cinnamon Chips

Serves: 5

Nutritional values per serving:

Calories: 312

Fat: 5.9 g

Carbohydrate: 59 g

Protein: 6.8 g

Ingredients

- 1 golden delicious apple, peeled, cored, cubed
- ½ pound strawberries
- 1 kiwi, peeled, cubed
- 4 ounces raspberries
- ½ tablespoon brown sugar
- 1 tablespoon white sugar
- 1 ½ tablespoons fruit preserve of your choice
- Butter-flavored cooking spray
- 5 flour tortillas (10 inches each)
- 1 tablespoon cinnamon sugar

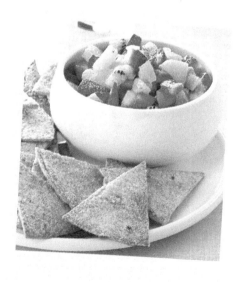

1. To make fruit salsa: Combine all the fruits, brown sugar, white sugar, and fruit preserve in a bowl.
2. Keep the bowl covered in the refrigerator until use.
3. To make cinnamon chips: Set the temperature of the oven to 350° F and preheat the oven.
4. Spray butter-flavored cooking spray over the top of the tortillas. Cut the tortillas into wedges.
5. Place the tortilla wedges on a large baking sheet. Use 2 baking sheets if necessary. Sprinkle cinnamon sugar on top
6. Place the baking sheet in the oven and set the timer for 8–10 minutes, in batches.
7. Cool completely and serve tortilla chips with fruit salsa.

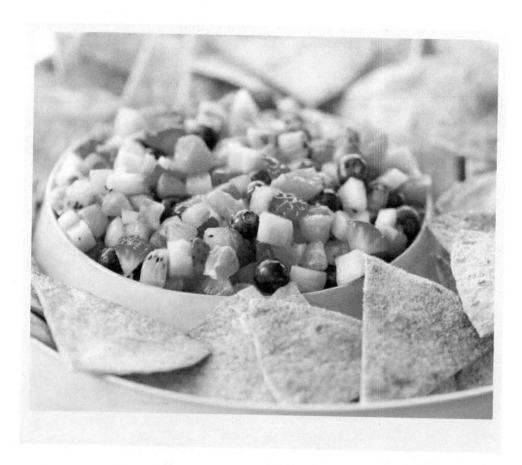

Rocky Road Parfaits

Serves: 8

Nutritional values per serving:

Calories: 243

Fat: 9 g

Carbohydrate: 34 g

Protein: 7 g

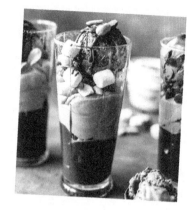

Ingredients

- 2 packages (4 serving sizes each)
  chocolate or chocolate fudge instant pudding mix
- 1 cup frozen whipped dessert topping, thawed
- ½ cup mini marshmallows
- ½ cup roasted, chopped unsalted peanuts
- 4 cups milk
- Chocolate curls to garnish (optional)

Directions

1. Follow the instructions given on the package of the pudding and make the pudding.
2. Add about 1 ½ cups of the prepared pudding to a bowl and add whipped topping. Fold until just combined.
3. Divide the remaining pudding equally into 8 parfait glasses. Spoon the whipped topping mixture on top. Keep it aside for about 10-15 minutes until it sets. Chill if desired.
4. Sprinkle peanuts, marshmallows, and chocolate curls on top and serve.

Chocolate Banana Cookies

Serves: 60

Nutritional values per serving:

Calories: 85

Fat: 3.4 g

Carbohydrate: 13.2 g

Protein: 1.2 g

Ingredients

- 2 cups white-whole wheat flour
- 1 teaspoon baking soda
- 2 teaspoons baking powder
- 1/8 teaspoon salt
- 1 medium banana, sliced
- 1 cup packed brown sugar
- 2 eggs
- 2 cups old-fashioned oats
- 6 tablespoons unsweetened cocoa powder
- 1 teaspoon ground cinnamon
- ½ cup canola oil
- 1 ½ cups confectioners' sugar
- 2 teaspoons vanilla extract
- 1 cup semi-sweet chocolate chips

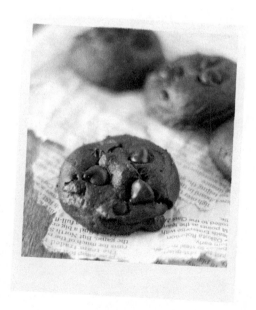

Directions

1. Set the temperature of the oven to 350° F and preheat the oven.
2. Prepare 2 to 3 large baking sheets by lining them with parchment paper.
3. Place banana slices in a bowl and mash them up with a fork until very smooth. Make sure there are no chunks in it.
4. Stir in oil, confectioners' sugar, brown sugar, vanilla, and eggs.
5. Combine flour, baking soda, baking powder, and salt in a bowl.
6. Add egg mixture into the flour mixture and stir until just combined. Add chocolate chips and oats and fold gently.
7. Take out a tablespoonful of the mixture and place it on the baking sheet. Repeat with the remaining mixture. Make sure to leave sufficient gaps between the cookies.
8. Press the cookies (to the desired thickness). Place the baking sheet in the oven and set the timer for 10 to 12 minutes or until they are golden brown around the edges.
9. Cook the remaining cookies in batches. Let them cool on the baking sheet for about 5 minutes.
10. Remove the cookies from the baking sheet and place them on a cooling rack.

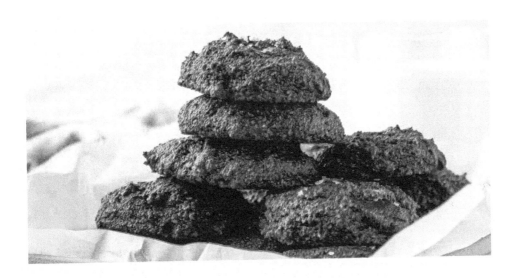

Chocolate Covered Strawberries

Serves: 15

Nutritional values per serving:

Calories: 40

Fat: 2 g

Carbohydrate: 4 g

Protein: 0.45 g

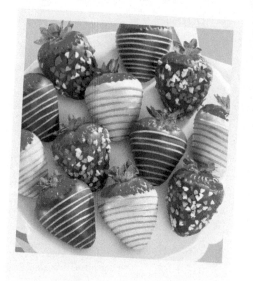

Ingredients

- 15 strawberries (1 pound)
- 5 ounces bittersweet or semi-sweet chocolate

Directions

1. Prepare a baking sheet by lining it with parchment paper or wax paper.
2. Melt chocolate in a double boiler or in a microwave.
3. Dip the strawberries held by the stem in melted chocolate and place them on the baking sheet.
4. Place the baking sheet in the refrigerator and chill until the chocolate sets over the strawberries.
5. Serve.

Conclusion

I want to thank you once again for choosing this book. I hope it proved to be an enjoyable and informative read.

Learning that you are pregnant for the first time is a life-changing experience. It comes with a slew of emotions that will leave you feeling excited one moment and panicking the next. This is extremely common and nothing to worry about. Dear first-time mama, this pregnancy will be an incredibly special time in your life. That said, it is also a time when you will be the recipient of unsolicited advice from different sources. Whether it is Reddit threads, social media, or a well-meaning neighbor, be prepared for advice about what you should and should not be doing. Therefore, you must not be overloaded by unhelpful prenatal information and instead, obtain the right information. This is where this book steps into the picture. It will act as your guide every step of the way.

In this book, you were introduced to all things associated with prenatal nutrition. Not just about the nutrients your body requires during pregnancy but after pregnancy as well. You were also introduced to a variety of foods that you should and should not eat for a healthy pregnancy. Consuming a healthy and well-balanced diet is not just needed for your health but for your baby as well. Growing a baby within your body is no easy feat. Therefore, focusing on the right nutrition is needed. The first step to shifting to a healthy diet is to understand the role of nutrition in your health. Your body requires different macro and micronutrients. Getting your daily dose of them is pivotal for your pregnancy and there are no shortcuts here. It's not just about the type of food you opt for, but the quality of ingredients also matters. Everything associated with nutrition throughout pregnancy was given in this book.

Now that you are equipped with the information you need about nutrition during and after pregnancy, it's time to implement the advice. The good news is that you don't have to look any further and spend time searching for pregnancy-friendly recipes. All the recipes you require for the different trimesters are given in this book. You simply need to take some time, create a meal plan, gather the required ingredients, and follow the simple instructions. These are the only steps you need to follow. Cooking has never been this easy before and you can forget about spending hours in the kitchen. All these recipes will cater to your daily nutritional requirements. So, you can rest easy knowing that you and your growing baby are obtaining the required nutrients in the right dosage.

So, what are you waiting for? There is no time like the present to get started, especially if you want to shift to earn a nutritious diet.

Thank you and all the best!

References

Bjarnadottir, A. (2020, August 13). 11 Foods and Beverages to Avoid During Pregnancy. Healthline. https://www.healthline.com/nutrition/11-foods-to-avoid-during-pregnancy#10.-Alcohol

Breastfeeding and your diet. (n.d.). Www.betterhealth.vic.gov.au. https://www.betterhealth.vic.gov.au/health/healthyliving/breastfeeding-and-your-diet

Hecht, A. (2002, May 27). Pregnancy and Prenatal Vitamins. WebMD; WebMD. https://www.webmd.com/baby/guide/prenatal-vitamins

How to Eat Well in Your Second Trimester of Pregnancy. (2018, December 18). Healthline. https://www.healthline.com/health/pregnancy/second-trimester-diet-nutrition#tips-for-healthy-eating

LisaG. (2019, April 7). 11 Common Pregnancy Diet Mistakes (And How to Avoid Them!). Birth Eat Love. https://www.birtheatlove.com/pregnancy-eating-mistakes/

Moss, M. (n.d.). What's the Right Portion Size When Pregnant? More. Retrieved July 2, 2022, from Https://www.more.com/lifestyle/whats-right-portion-size-when-pregnant/

Nierenberg, C., & Wild, S. (2021, April 24). Pregnancy Diet & Nutrition: What to Eat, What Not to Eat. Livescience.com. https://www.livescience.com/45090-pregnancy-diet.html#section-foods-to-eat

Prenatal vitamins: Why they matter, how to choose. (2020, November 13). Mayo Clinic. https://www.mayoclinic.org/healthy-lifestyle/pregnancy-week-by-week/basics/healthy-pregnancy/hlv-20049471

Made in the USA
Las Vegas, NV
04 October 2024

96280062R00072